DATE DUE

OCT 27 1993	
APR 2 8	
NOV 15 1995	
NOV 29 199:	
MAR 1 0 1999	

BRODART   Cat. No. 23-221

CONTEMPORARY ISSUES
IN PAEDIATRIC ETHICS

Edited by

Michael M. Burgess

and

Brian E. Woodrow

The Edwin Mellen Press
Lewiston/Queenston/Lampeter

Library of Congress Cataloging-in-Publication Data

This volume has been registered with The Library of Congress.

Co-sponsored by Alberta Children's Hospital Child Health Centre, Calgary, Alberta

ISBN 0-7734-9673-4

A CIP catalog record for this book
is available from the British Library.

The Edwin Mellen Press
Box 450
Lewiston, New York
USA 14092

The Edwin Mellen Press
Box 67
Queenston, Ontario
CANADA L0S 1L0

The Edwin Mellen Press, Ltd.
Lampeter, Dyfed, Wales
UNITED KINGDOM SA48 7DY

Printed in the United States of America

DEDICATION

In the fog of ignorance, uncertainty, ambiguity and perplexity that permeates decision making about infants and children, this beacon serves to keep the party of responsible adults focused: seeking to do that which might be in the child's best interests.

William G. Bartholome

TABLE OF CONTENTS

Preface

The incredible scientific and medical advances, economic constraints and conflicting human values in our society have created a biomedical revolution. How should we make our choices when faced with moral dilemmas in the delivery of health care to paediatric patients and their families? The topics addressed in this collection are becoming increasingly familiar to paediatric health care practitioners and consumers.

In 1985, at the Alberta Children's Hospital Child Health Centre, a biomedical ethics planning group was founded to respond to the moral problems confronting practitioners and parents. This group considered consultation and education as two practical approaches, and decided to give priority to education. One of the educational projects was a conference, drawing upon international scholarship with a focus on practical problems of both local and universal interest. Although the faculty were professional philosophers, theologians, physicians and lawyers, the participants included a wide range of health care practitioners, parents and the public. The practical, non-technical and interdisciplinary flavour of the conference is reflected in the content and style of these essays, which are edited versions of the conference presentations.

In the first of these papers, David Ost, philosopher and former director of Old Dominion University's Institute of Applied Ethics, surveys the range and complexities of ethical issues in paediatric care.

William Bartholome, a paediatrician with a graduate degree in Theology and professor of History and Philosophy of Medicine at the University of Kansas Medical Center, discusses decisions to withhold or withdraw care. Bartholome suggests that such decisions must be based on the child's best interests. He rejects the notion of parental or guardian "proxy consent," suggesting instead that informed parental permission be supported with the requirement of the child-patient's assent and agreement from "the circle of primary decision-makers" including the nursing care staff. If this procedure fails, a hospital ethics committee should serve as a "backup" system.

Terry Ackerman, philosopher and director of the Program on Human Values and Ethics at the University of Tennessee Center for the Health Sciences, asks whether children have a moral right to receive innovative lifesaving treatment at society's expense. Although he does not establish such a moral right, Ackerman does show that arguments against this right fail, and that the medically worse off children "have a strong moral claim against the resources of a society."

Michael Burgess, a philosopher and professor of bioethics for the Faculty of Medicine and the Humanities Institute at the University of Calgary, addresses the issues arising in health care from an increased awareness of the range of variation in minors' maturity. Emphasizing individualized assessment and relationships as critical elements which replace age definitions of competency and consent, Burgess suggests that children ought always to be involved in their care. This involvement may be through efforts to emotionally support and avoid unnecessary fear and pain, through explanation, asking permission or honouring full informed consent requirements.

Susan Sherwin, philosopher and chair of the philosophy department at Dalhousie University in Halifax, criticizes the notion of non-treatment and non-compliance as neglect for its assumption of the medical profession's authority to determine what are the best interests for children. Sherwin suggests that transfer of parental authority is only appropriate in the presence of authoritative technical information establishing the child's best medical interests, and that the accusation of neglect must be independently established on evidence that the parents are not sufficiently interested in the child's welfare. A focus on neglect undermines trust as the basis for good, therapeutic relationships.

Herbert O'Driscoll, poet, theologian, and rector of Christ Church in Calgary, summarizes and synthesizes the content of the previous discussions. O'Driscoll sets the issues in a larger context, identifies common values and suggests some exciting future developments.

Although the editors acknowledge full responsibility for errors in organization and summary, the conference on May 13 and 14, 1987 was only possible because of the support and assistance of many people and institutions. The Alberta Children's Hospital Child Health Centre (ACHCHC), the Alberta Heritage Foundation for Medical Research, Health and Welfare Canada and the University of Calgary's Special Projects Fund all gave financial support for the conference, with additional support for publication of this volume from the ACHCHC. Robert Innes and Jean Roberts gave administrative support, Rita Pugh and Gail Graham gave patient and indispensable secretarial assistance, and Florence Kubinec, Nursing Co-ordinator for Education and Quality Assurance, and Michael McKernan, Mental Health Social Worker, were on the planning committee, which laid the groundwork for the conference and this book. All of the above people were granted time for their efforts by the ACHCHC. Laurie Bennie organized the generous volunteer support of the ACHCHC Community Advisory Committee, without which the conference would have been impossible. Dr. T. D. Kinsella, Assistant Dean (Medical Bioethics) at the University of Calgary, chaired the evening session and panel discussion. Greta Cowx, Stella Massey-Hicks and Donna Wong typed and revised the manuscript. To all these, and unmentioned others, we express our most sincere gratitude.

Michael Burgess
Brian Woodrow

Bioethics and Paediatrics

David Ost

"The history of childhood," wrote Lloyd DeMause (1974), "is a nightmare from which we have only recently begun to awaken." From a contemporary perspective, that history is nightmarish indeed, recounting a litany of physical abuse ranging from regular beatings to the killing of children, either actively or by abandonment, and widely practiced in both the East and West. Children were often regarded as property, owned by their parents like other assets – and of course liabilities – who could be used in the fields if one were a peasant, or to cement political and/or economic relationships if one were an aristocrat or a merchant. The concept of "the good of the child" was of secondary importance, if it was considered at all. Notice, for example, the concept of filial gratitude. You have all heard the quotation, I am sure, "how sharper than a serpent's tooth it is, to have a thankless child" (Shakespeare, I:4). Such a concept can only make coherent sense if providing a good life for one's children is regarded as supererogatory, that is, above and beyond the call of parental duty. We are not normally grateful to others for fulfilling their obligations toward us. We quite legitimately expect that they will do that. Gratitude is an appropriate response only for a gift freely given, not for an obligation that one must, morally, fulfill.

While our current normative attitudes toward children form a remarkable contrast to those that we can cull from our cultural history, we commonly take it to be the case that we have at least as strong moral obligations to children generally as we do to adults, and that we have especially strong ones, as parents, to our own children. At law, we prohibit parents from taking some actions with respect to their children and we hold them seriously accountable for failing to provide for their children a number of important services. We also place upon some professional groups, health care professionals among them, a positive duty to report parental transgressions against, or neglect of, their children. The foundational concern served by these injunctions, both active and passive, is the concept of the best interest of the child in his or her own right. But it is worth keeping in mind the lesson of history, that currency of an attitude is no guarantee of its ethical soundness. This attitude may be a psychological fact about us, but we would need to examine its ethical underpinnings. Do we indeed have such obligations to children? And if so what is their content and limits?

The Moral Status of the Child

Like the concept of childhood itself, a concept with fuzzy edges, the moral status of the child is not a clearly settled issue. The ordinary focal concept of moral status in ethics is the concept of a "person." "Person," here, is a technical term, identifying an entity which is first of all capable of deliberating rationally over alternative courses of action, and, second, capable of freely and voluntarily choosing among those alternatives; that is, a rational, free, self-determining agent. Only such agents, it is held by Immanuel Kant among others, are capable of assuming the burdens that morality requires, only such agents can be the subjects of moral obligations, only such agents (perhaps more importantly for our purposes) can be the bearers of rights. Children, particularly young children, do not possess these qualities of rational self-determination. Just as it would be foolish of us to expect of children a recognition of their moral obligations, as we do of adults, or to hold them accountable for failing to meet such obligations, as we also do in the case of adults, it would be equally as foolish to treat them as bearers of rights in the adult sense. Where adults may, for example, as a matter of right, refuse medical treatment, the refusal by a four-year-old of an antibiotic injection is not the assertion of a right that must be respected, but rather the expression of a preference which may be, and is, regularly overridden in the child's best interest. On such a view, children have no rights intrinsically and one owes no obligations to children directly.

One may, however, owe obligations to other moral agents about children. Thus, for example, an injury to a child can be a moral wrong, however it is not a moral wrong to the child, but rather to other moral agents, for example parents, who have a proprietary interest in the child. Now there is obviously very little in this focal approach to the moral status of children that suggests a plausible conceptual foundation for our contemporary attitudes. We recognize that children are among the class of those who are incompetent to function as moral agents, but we do not hold that children are thus without moral status in and of themselves. Yet, how may we justify this judgment?

Perhaps one might hold, as H. Tristram Engelhardt, Jr. does, that while children are not persons in the strict sense that I have just outlined, they may be recognized as persons in a secondary and derivative sense. Engelhardt says:

> Young children live as persons in and through the care of those who are responsible for them, and those responsible for them exercise the children's rights on their behalf. In this sense, children belong to families in ways that most adults do not. As social entities, children exist in and through their families. (Engelhardt, 1975)

Here, while rights are not something children intrinsically possess, they are at least imputed to children by virtue of the child's ability to function in a particular social role: the role of "child." Thus, for social purposes, we treat children as if they were persons although we recognize that intrinsically they are not.

Clearly, on this view, the rights children possess are solely the rights we, as adult members of a society, agree to grant them. But such an agreement would constitute a social choice rather than a moral compulsion. If we so choose, we might grant them no rights at all. Engelhardt is quite frank about the implications of his position. It would be morally permissible actively to kill very young children, if it were desirable on other grounds to do so, and if doing so would not result in erosion of the social role of "child" generally.

Alternatively, one might focus on the potentiality of children to become adult persons. On this view, one's treatment of children is constrained by obligations to the person the child will become. Thus our obligations to children now are based upon the perception that the events of childhood shape or warp the adult, crippling or incapacitating him physically or psychologically. The moral wrong here, it should be stressed, is again not a wrong directly to the child, but rather to the adult he will become. Thus, were there no chance that the child would in fact become an adult (one might think here of the presence of terminal illness), then it would seem that no act perpetrated on such a child would constitute a moral wrong.

Obviously, none of the approaches just outlined does justice to our moral intuitions about the treatment of children, nor certainly to the strength and depth of those intuitions. We might well argue by contrast that these conceptions of moral status are perhaps too constrictive, that children have another distinctive property which they share in common with adults and with at least higher-level animals, and that is the ability to suffer (Singer, 1975). These are explicitly utilitarian arguments whose main principle is the maximization of happiness and the minimization of suffering, for those entities capable of achieving happiness or of being subject to suffering. Clearly, one need not be a rational free agent, on this view, to count morally. Kittens, for example, are surely not rational, free agents, but we would not hold that torturing kittens for enjoyment or for idle curiosity is entirely morally neutral. Even where there is no question of violating the interests of other moral agents, we should hold that the infliction of unjustified suffering on the kitten is a wrong to the kitten directly. If, as these philosophers maintain, we have a moral duty to refrain from the infliction of unjustified suffering upon others and to relieve the suffering of others even where those others cannot qualify as competent moral agents, then it may be precisely this capacity for suffering which calls forth our obligations toward children.

Thus, on this basis, one might observe that minimally and in a *prima facie* way, parents have an obligation toward their children to minimize their suffering and that we as a society have similar obligations to intervene in situations, even familial situations, in which unnecessary or unjustified suffering is produced. Now I have suggested that this is a *prima facie*

obligation, not an absolute one; perhaps time will not permit the sketching of its restrictions or limits, and these may be many. One might note, however, two points. First, that something like this principle can be seen as the foundation for the *parens patriae* function of the state, that function in terms of which the state serves as guardian of the best interests of those who are incompetent to assess those interests or to secure freedom from harm on their own behalf. The second is that parental obligations are particularly powerful ones. Even the wanted child, for example, is never initially wanted in his or her own full particularity, for he or she does not yet exist as a possible object of desire. With respect to my daughter, for example, when my wife and I conceived the child, we intended to conceive a child but not the child we actually produced. The child is an entity brought into being not to satisfy its own interests, for it as yet has none, but to satisfy an interest of the parents. In satisfying their own interests, parents have, in fact, enabled, for the resulting child, the joys of life, but by the same act they have also enabled the pain and suffering that life inevitably brings. Thus we charge parents with especially powerful obligations of protection and nurturance of those entities they have endowed with the mixed blessing of existence. For the most part, the state delegates the ability to decide the best interests of incompetents, like children, to their nearest relatives on the presumption that these persons are best situated physically, emotionally and morally to make best-interest assessments. Parents are also charged with both the right and the obligation to give informed consent for the medical treatment of their children, as well as rights to make a wide variety of decisions on their children's behalf, and it is here that health care professionals bear a special responsibility.

The Child as a Patient

Recognizing the incompetence of children to decide their own future course and the special obligations of parents with regard to their children, paediatric medicine also operates under the presumption of best interests, that is, that parents have both the right and the obligation to choose the course of action which they judge to be in the best interest of their child. Given that the child is incompetent to consent to his or her own medical treatment and that others must consent on the child's behalf, the doctrine of informed consent instructs us to turn to the parents for the consent procedure.

It is sometimes startling to health care professionals to hear the claim that patients do not exist, especially coming from a philosopher whose claim sounds like the prelude to an abstruse exercise in metaphysics, but my intent in making this claim is much more prosaic. The term "patient" identifies a social role which, from time to time in their lives, individuals may play. Normally, this observation serves as a prelude to a discussion of moral pitfalls of reducing the individual's interests as a person to his or her medical interests as a patient, that is, a discussion of the temptations of medical paternalism; but here I want to use this observation in a somewhat different way. The relationship between a physician and a patient, the relationship, that is, on which all other health care professional/patient relationships are modeled, is a social role relationship, and one which carries with it role-generated obligations. The physician, for example, is obligated to act in the best interests of the patient's health. The person fulfilling the social role of patient may well choose an alternative course of action, relieving the professional of this responsibility, as is the case, for example, when a competent patient declines a recommended medical intervention.

But it is important to say that this obligation is not owed to a particular person, as such, by virtue of the person's possession of the qualities of personhood. It is owed rather, in and through the medical relationship, to the occupant of the social role "patient." Thus, for example, when the occupant of that social role is a small child, even though parents are charged with both the right and the obligation of informed consent on the child's behalf, a parental refusal of treatment, or request for one, does not definitively settle the question of professional obligation to one's patient. In the prosaic case, for example, in which parents request that antibiotics be prescribed for their child's self-limiting viral infection, and where the professional's best clinical judgment is that treatment with antibiotics will have at best marginal benefit and some potential risk for his patient's health, the professional may be construed to have an obligation to resist acceding to that request. The parental right to informed consent does not eliminate or replace the health care professional's obligation to the patient. Such a consideration may, at times, entail that the professional become an advocate for the interests of the child.

What I have said so far indicates that while there is a generalized presumption in favour of respecting decisions made by parents with regard to their children, health care professionals, by virtue of their obligations to their patients, have a special obligation to determine whether there are serious reasons for questioning or overriding this presumption. What might such reasons look like?

In one classic sort of case, a child is born with Down's syndrome and an esophageal fistula, whose presence precludes feeding. The parents refuse treatment for the fistula, though it is easily correctable surgically. Other statements made by the parents at this time suggest that their refusal of treatment is motivated less by consideration of the best interest of the child than by their own interest in not bearing the burden of care for a defective child. In this sort of instance, one has grounds for questioning whether parents are even seeking to fulfill their obligation of care for their child. In another sort of case, a child is brought to the emergency room by ambulance after collapsing in school. She is diagnosed as having acute appendicitis for which surgery is urgently needed. Her parents, who have rushed to the hospital after notification by the school, refuse surgery. They assert that they are members of a religious group which relies upon the healing power of prayer and a consent to medical treatment on their part would not only be a serious sin for them, their doctrine also holds that it would prevent their daughter from entering into eternal life should she die. Here, the medical staff are faced with parents whose sincere belief that they are in fact acting in the best interest of their daughter in the long term is unquestionable, but on the analysis of the professional obligation to their patient that has just been suggested, they may be obliged to seek a court order compelling treatment.

The point behind these cases is not that the health care professional is the final arbiter of the best interests of the child; it is, rather, that by virtue of the social role obligations of the professional, he or she may be morally compelled to question parental rights of choice regarding children and to carry this questioning into a wider public arena, namely the courts, on at least some occasions, and this compulsion holds despite the appeal, as in the last case, to sincere religious conviction. Though parents are guaranteed a legal right under the U.S. Constitution, and the Canadian Charter of Rights and Freedoms, to religious freedom, and a right to raise their children in accordance with the tenets of that religion, the courts in the U.S. have regularly held that parents may not subject their children to serious risks to health and welfare even where these are risks the parents themselves are quite willing to undertake for religious reasons. While court cases have supported, for example, the refusal of life-saving blood transfusions on the part of adult Jehovah's Witnesses, they have generally tended to order such transfusions for the minor children of Jehovah's Witnesses.

Some years ago, the members of a small religious sect in Brooklyn, New York, were brought to trial on the charge that they had beaten to death, with baseball bats, the fourteen-year-old daughter of one of their members. In their defense, the group argued that they had been following the doctrine of their religion, acting in the girl's best interest, for she had been possessed by the devil, and their actions had been aimed at saving her soul by beating the devil from her body. It was surely tragic that she had died in this process, but there had been no intent on their part to kill her. From their point of view and in the words of one of my colleagues, her death then seems, from their perspective, as unfortunate but not immoral. Religious claims of this sort are particularly troublesome, for while we seek to protect children from suffering, we seek also to protect the rights of adults. However, while religious freedom is a fundamental freedom, like the freedom of parents to raise their children as they see fit, it cannot be an unrestricted freedom. Treatment of children which we should condemn, when undertaken for other motivations, is treatment that the cloak of religious freedom ought not, by itself, to justify. If it is wrong to beat a child with a baseball bat for fun, or for purposes of discipline, or for any other reason, then the claim of religious motivation does not alter the moral quality of the act.

Given that health care professionals have obligations to children as patients, the fairly simple articulation of these principles does not, by itself, resolve the sorts of complex issues that can arise in the context of the delivery of health care. It is to at least two of these issues that I should like now to turn. Children's participation in decisions will be addressed in somewhat greater detail by William Bartholome and Michael Burgess. I should begin, then, with the issue of child abuse.

Child Abuse

There is perhaps no issue which excites greater pathos or public outrage than the abuse of children. The image of an adult inflicting injury upon a small child, powerless in its vulnerability, is calculated to evoke both horror and anger. It is a fundamental violation of our ingrained social attitude that the only morally defensible sorts of confrontation are those which can occur among relative equals. Today we recognize at least three major categories of child abuse. The first is, of course, the battered child. One news story in Virginia focused on a child, now two years of age, who had suffered severe brain damage. His head had been smashed so forcefully against the floor of his playpen that the metal supports beneath the floor had been bent. The mother and her boyfriend disclaimed any knowledge of how this had occurred, indicating that they had both left the house for "just a few minutes" and returned to find the child injured. The second category is the sexually abused child. A flurry of new reports in the United States over the past two years has focused on the discovery of sexual abuse of children at several day-care centres in different parts of the country. The growth of day care as part of contemporary life, coupled with inadequate state regulation of such centres and their personnel, suggest that this problem is likely to get significantly worse before it gets any better. At the same time we have become more highly conscious of the problem of incest and sexual abuse of children by other family members. We have recognized that the incidence of such abuse is far more widespread than we might have imagined. The third category is that of the neglected child. Newspapers also carry frequent stories of so-called "latchkey children," small children left alone at home to fend for themselves while adults responsible for their care are at work. Another account, for example, in a newspaper in the United States detailed the case of two children, ages two and four, who died as a result of having been locked in a car, in a hot climate, for a twenty-four hour period.

There is a fourth category, emotional or psychological abuse, which is generally noted by workers in child and family studies, but about which others have raised serious definitional problems. When abuse is extended to include emotional injury, it is sometimes argued, the door is opened for zealous professionals to intervene punitively in virtually any parent-child relationship. On the other hand, however, emotional injury to a child can be equally as serious, as crippling, and as long term as any physical injury. Part of the problem is that we have no clear-cut understanding of what constitutes abuse. Certainly, in the three categories that I have listed, extreme cases like those described are fairly obvious, but what of corporal punishment, or even caning, still widely used by parents as a disciplinary measure, and in the United States, at least, legally sanctioned in the schools? Is this a form of battery? What of the standard practiced by nursemaids in some European countries of quieting a crying child by fondling its genitalia? Does this constitute sexual abuse?

Serious persons concerned about the problem of child abuse recommend listening very carefully to children when they make such reports, but this may not be as easy as it sounds. The child lives in a world in which the demarcation between reality and fantasy is not clear-cut, and this problem is particularly acute in cases of suspected sexual abuse without decisive physiological confirmation. It is less problematic in cases of battery or neglect where the child's condition bears witness to the existence of the problem. Similarly, young children have no basis for comparison of their situation with that of others and can often see their own situation only through the eyes of their parents, assuming, in fact, the guilt imputed to them. ("Yes, my daddy or mommy hit me, but I was being very bad.") The professional, suspecting child abuse, is often faced with a situation for which he or she is completely untrained, sorting out the realities of a home situation from conflicting and highly hedged reports. One might contend, then, that by virtue of obligations to the patient, the professional ought, if anything, to err on the side of patient protection and report even doubtful cases of abuse on the theory that others that are appropriately trained will be able to sort out the facts.

But there is a problem here as well. In many instances, the response of social services agencies to reports of child abuse is a swift one. The child is immediately removed from the home while investigation of the charge is in progress. If the charge is a false one, and some seventy-five percent of such charges are generally regarded as unfounded, the effects on parents can be devastating. To be accused of abusing one's child, to have one's children wrenched from one by a state agency and placed in the care of strangers, to be the subjects of minute scrutiny and questioning, are all traumatic enough. But the social consequences, ostracism and suspicion by one's neighbours, destruction of careers and the termination of employment which may follow from public knowledge that such an investigation is even in progress, and threatening or abusive telephone calls from anonymous parties, may be catastrophic to the family as a whole. Further, even if the charges are true, there is also the possibility that a change in custody may be more harmful to the child than an admittedly unsatisfactory home situation. Considerations such as these suggest that an uncritical acceptance of the rule, "when in doubt, report," may be ill-considered. They also suggest that while the consequences to the professional may end with his or her report, the responsibility for those consequences to others may not. There is, in effect, no substitute for careful thought, whether one reports or does not report child abuse.

Personhood

Another set of issues concerns the progressive development of children into adulthood. We have seen that small children, at least, are members of the class of incompetents, insofar as they lack the crucial two prerequisites for rational free agency, "personhood" in the strict sense, and thus others are called upon to make best-interest assessments on their behalf. But children not only have the potential to become persons in their own right; in the natural course of events, they will come to actualize that potential, and acquire the decision-making rights that come with that actualization. The key question becomes, at what point can children be said to have acquired that status and those rights?

The classic philosophical way of characterizing rational free agents is to ascribe to them the quality of autonomy, the capability of self-determination, and the classic difficulty is that autonomy is not a monolithic concept but a much more complex phenomenon. That adults generally possess this moral status does not entail that all their acts are the product of autonomous deliberation, nor does it entail that adults are perfectly autonomous in all areas of their lives at all times. Autonomy in the adult admits of degrees; thus we talk of "diminished autonomy" with respect to some sorts of patients. It admits of departments; that one is autonomous, for example, in managing one's business affairs does not entail that one is autonomous in choosing one's medical treatment. It admits even of questions about bare presence. A febrile patient drifting in and out of delirium is sometimes autonomous, sometimes not. Autonomy is not a quality which is acquired "whole cloth" and overnight.

The older child is an entity on the way to adult autonomy, and like any other traveller on a journey, he is no longer at his point of origin and not yet at his destination. No longer clearly non-autonomous, he is not yet able to claim all his rights as his own. Such a child is, however, capable of filling the social role of patient rather more amply than the infant or the young child is; that is, he is capable of understanding, at least in a simplified way, the importance of treatment and the course that treatment will follow. It is here that the concept of assent becomes operative.

If one of the obligations of health care professionals to their patients is captured in the phrase "respect for persons," then such respect is due to the extent that personhood is present, that is, respect for autonomous self-determination is owed to an entity whose moral dimensions now transcend the simple ability to occupy the social role of patient. Such an observation suggests two points with respect to informed consent. First, that information is owed to the patient, and, where the patient is capable of being informed in even the most rudimentary fashion, that obligation is not discharged by merely informing even legitimate proxy decision-makers alone; and, second, where the occupant of the social role, patient, is capable of forming and expressing a best interest judgment, that judgment may not simply be ignored, but requires consideration. This latter point does not mean that the judgments of minors, even mature ones, are ultimately decisive. Informed consent is a right of autonomous patients, but its character as a burden ought not to be ignored. Individuals who choose freely and autonomously and whose choices must be respected, assume, along with those choices, their consequences, both positive and negative. To assume that a choice is autonomous simply because it is articulated, making that assumption in circumstances that render autonomy at least questionable, is to risk imposing upon the patient articulating the choice a set of consequences he might not choose to accept were he fully autonomous.

Giving the judgments of older children consideration entails attending to their expressed choices, and accommodating those choices to the extent possible within the limits of the patient's best interests. Thus, while one cannot rely for informed consent upon the older child, one has the obligation to secure informed assent and to accommodate demurrers where possible. A further point is important here. Autonomy is a moral concept; competence, on the other hand, is generally a medico-legal one. For the most part, although not necessarily always, those who fail to meet the requirements of competence will fail also to meet the criteria of autonomy, and the assent of the child will fulfill one's obligation. But the dimension of autonomy most directly important to health care professionals is the much narrower concept of competence to consent to treatment, and it is at least possible that some older children will in fact be capable of giving informed consent to treatment on their own behalf. Where the judgments of such children conflict with those of their parents, health care professionals are faced with a serious dilemma. To respect the choice of the parents is to deny the child the moral right to decide his own fate, a right to which his moral status entitles him. The obligation of respect for persons here, in their social role of patient, would suggest that the balance should fall on the side of patient, calling for support and advocacy by health care professionals of the patient's choice.

Well, what have we seen? We have seen, first, that there is a plausible foundation for the claim that we owe obligations to children directly and not only through intermediaries. Based upon the capacity of children, like adults, to suffer, we have seen that the holders of a variety of social roles bear special obligations, by virtue of those roles, to relieve the suffering and promote the best interests of children, in particular the social roles of parents and health care professionals. The paediatric relationship manifests three different roles: the role of parents, the role of the patient, and the role of the health care professional. We have explored briefly, but not, I hope, without usefulness, some of the potential ethical conflicts that can arise in that complex relationship.

REFERENCES

DeMause, Lloyd. 1974. *A History of Childhood.* New York: Psycho-history Press.

Engelhardt, Jr., H. T. 1975. Ethical Issues in Aiding in the Death of Young Children. *Beneficent Euthanasia*, edited by Marvin Kohl. Buffalo, N. Y.: Prometheus Books. History Press.

Shakespeare, William. *King Lear.* Act. I, Scene 4: 277-278.

Singer, Peter. 1975. *Animal Liberation.* New York: Random House.

Withholding/Withdrawing Life-Sustaining Treatment

William G. Bartholome

Introduction

Most of the work that has been done on the ethical issues involved in decisions to withhold or withdraw life-sustaining treatment in paediatrics has focused on the care of infants (Weir, 1984; Murray and Caplan, 1985). Our public dialogue has focused almost exclusively on infants who were physically and/or mentally handicapped and in need of treatment for a life-threatening condition. In this paper I will attempt to expand the range of concerns to include consideration of the ethical issues involved when such decisions involve older children, adolescents and young adults.

The paper is basically a complex argument which focuses on how I think these decisions ought to be made. I use the word "ought" in this context advisedly since the position I will outline may not be the ethical way of making withholding/withdrawal decisions. I am not attempting to argue that this is the only way or even the best way to go about making these complex and difficult decisions. It represents, I hope, a way of making such decisions that is arguably ethical, i.e., a method that reflects a sensitivity to the nature of these decisions; that reflects a commitment to the interests of the child/patient; and, which can be defended using the language and concepts of ethics.

The Decision: What is at Stake?

To begin with I think it is critically important that we look at the kind of decision we are considering; the nature of the decision. I would argue that there are at least two fundamental ways of looking at decisions to withhold or withdraw life-sustaining treatment. First, in an important respect we are considering a decision to deprive an infant or child of his/her life. Granted that we will not know at the point of making the decision that the child will die, but we will know that this is the expected or foreseeable outcome. Decisions to deprive an individual of his/her life are decisions that societies generally regard as ones in which extreme caution, meticulous deliberation, "due process," and fair procedure are called for because of what is at stake. Life is regarded as not only a fundamental interest of human beings, but as a fundamental moral and legal entitlement or right. Although some consider it controversial (Melden, 1980), in this society, infants and children have or possess this fundamental legal and moral entitlement, i.e., the right to life. There is also in our thinking about life the idea that, in an important sense, life is the most basic good of all. It is hard to imagine an individual having or enjoying goods, enjoying what life has to offer both in the sense of moral and non-moral goods unless he/she is (or has been) alive. If we are to concern ourselves with any good or goods we must attend to this most basic, constitutive ingredient called life or existence.

Yet, from a different and equally important perspective we must not allow this consideration of what is at stake in such decisions to intimidate us. In an important sense such decisions challenge us to deal with the task of allowing infants and children to die; allowing death to come to them in spite of how threatening such an idea is to our conception of ourselves, of reality, of God. It is difficult, if not impossible, to have a stable worldview, a conception of "what's it all about?", a conception of God in which we can easily fit the reality of dying babies and children. So, even though we are talking about trading off this tremendously valuable thing called life, we are also dealing with something that is a very serious responsibility of health care providers and parents in caring for infants/children. These decisions involve a conscious, deliberate choice to not use or to discontinue the use of knowledge and technology that could be used and allowing the infant or child to die. It involves the very difficult task of "only caring" as Paul Ramsey has called it (Ramsey, 1970: 113-157). It involves, if you prefer the metaphors, the notion of release or relief which Elizabeth Kubler-Ross called to our attention (Kubler-Ross, 1975). It is the idea that here is a task for us as health care providers and parents that may well be from both a psychological and a moral standpoint one of the most challenging tasks we face. We must not be scared off by what is at stake here. If we cannot or will not "face the music" the price will be paid by an imperiled, critically ill infant or child.

What Kind of Decision is This?

I would next call attention to what may well be the most fundamental claim of my presentation. It is what might be referred to as the "take home message." The claim is that the decision to withhold or withdraw life-sustaining care is most fundamentally an ethical or moral or, if you like, human decision regarding the appropriate utilization of the knowledge and technology of health care professionals. Such a decision is not most fundamentally a medical decision, i.e., one to be decided by medical professionals on the basis of what is medically indicated or medically beneficial. Nor is it most fundamentally a nursing decision, i.e., one to be made by nursing professionals on the basis of what is indicated from the nursing assessment, diagnosis or plan. Although such a decision obviously involves these (and other) professionals and their knowledge and expertise, it is in a very fundamental sense a paradigm case of an ethical decision. The implications of that claim are broad and significant. It means no one can claim the expertise to make such a decision on the basis of their professional knowledge or experience (Veatch, 1981: 79-109). It means that no one individual can claim by virtue of his or her professional role the authority or the right to make such a decision. In fact one of the central themes in the contemporary debate about the ethical and legal rights of patients has been the idea that the patient has a crucial and indispensable role to play in making such decisions (Katz, 1984). As you will see, this claim is the foundation on which my entire argument about the ethical requirement for shared responsibility for making such decisions rests.

"Proxy Consent" and the Role of Parents/Guardians

As we begin it is important that we examine the set of questions that relate to the appropriate role and responsibility of parents in making such decisions. I would like to begin with a critical examination of the concept of "proxy consent." When I first got involved in the study of paediatric medical ethics through my involvement with the now infamous "Hopkins Case" in 1971 it was this issue that got my attention (Kennedy Foundation, 1971). It was the use of this concept that allowed the parents in that case to decide that they not only did not want to parent a child with Down's syndrome, but that a particular child with Down's syndrome was to be allowed to die. The health care professionals and the hospital involved in that case essentially washed their hands of all responsibility to that infant on the basis that they believed that the parents had the right of proxy consent; that they had the right to make this decision. In the 1970's it may have been possible to argue that the concept of "proxy consent" represented an understandable, even excusable, misunderstanding or misuse of what was coming to be called "informed consent" (Bartholome, 1982). In the 1980's it is no longer understandable or excusable. I think we need to explode the myth of proxy consent. We need to get rid of this dangerous concept and to replace it with a more appropriate way of talking about the role of parents in making these decisions.

Why is that? What is it about the concept of consent and this idea of "proxy consent" that require this reformulation? First, I think it is very important to understand something of the evolution of this concept (Faden and Beauchamp, 1986). Although this concept was born as a legal doctrine and requirement, it has been incorporated into our fundamental thinking about ethical issues in medicine and health care. It calls attention to an issue of fundamental importance that had been totally disregarded in the tradition of medical ethics. It calls attention to the idea that decision-making in the context of health care should be a joint endeavour. It should be one in which the patient has a voice and is not simply passive, accepting, obedient and compliant. This evolving doctrine calls attention to the values of knowledge and of freedom of liberty.

The ethical principle on which it is based is that of respect, respect for others. Often it is expressed as the concept of the respect for persons;

respect for the patient as a person. I have problems with the use of the concept of persons in this context since the concept has been co-opted by philosophers and used to refer to what they call "autonomous, rational agents" (Engelhardt, 1986: 104-109). I have never met one of those (and hope I never do!). I would rather use the concept of person in a much older, more traditional way; namely, that of a member of the human community: "one of us," if you like, a shorthand way of talking about persons (O'Donovan, 1984: 49-67). This principle of "respect for the patient as one of us" gives rise to the professional's duty of veracity. We are required not to lie to patients; not to deceive; to correct misconceptions and to disclose what is "really" going on. We are required to be honest; to be truthful; to honour the patient's right to know, the right to the truth, the whole truth. The principle of respect also calls attention to the idea that they, like us, are self-governing; that they are the primary guardians and caretakers of their health. As such, they should have the freedom to choose without coercion what they see as "the right," "the good" for them. Often this freedom is referred to as the right of self-determination. Thus, the concept of informed consent can have a tremendously liberating and empowering effect on the patient in the health care context and serves as an important corrective on the highly paternalistic nature of traditional professional ethics.

However, the concept has a serious problem at its core. The concept of consent is inherently ambiguous. It is used to refer to two very different kinds of judgments. We use it, I think most fundamentally and most accurately, to describe judgments made about self; as a statement about one's self. Literally translated, consent means "to feel, see or sense with"; consent means "I see it that way; what you propose fits me and my understanding of myself; my feelings; my thoughts; my goals." However, consent is also interpreted as being a statement about what is being proposed; what course of action is being recommended by the professional. It is in this second sense that our understanding of consent has led to the misleading notion that it can be done by proxy; that someone other than the patient can make a judgment about what is being proposed.

Aside from this fundamental ambiguity in the concept, additional problems were introduced when the concept was quickly incorporated into the discourse of rights. Since we have come to believe that the only way to insure that an ethical issue is given appropriate consideration is to express it in the legalistic language of rights, the concept of informed consent has come to be framed in the language of rights. By the early 1980's we had enshrined in our thinking the idea that patients have both the ethical and the legal right to consent or to refuse consent to any intervention proposed by the health care professional. This, like all rights, became what might be called a "trump card" in the dialogue about what "ought" to be done in the clinical context. Another way of thinking about it is to use the metaphor of a train. The train represents the momentum of the health care enterprise: the health care professional examines the patient, establishes the diagnosis, undertakes diagnostic studies and formulates a plan of action. Yet the patient holds the switch and can cause the entire health care team and the momentum of the entire enterprise to come to a screeching halt by simply saying the little word that two- and three-year-olds love so dearly, namely "NO!" This right puts ultimate power and control (at least theoretically) squarely in the hands of the patient.

So, what of "consent by proxy"? My argument is that this evolution renders the concept unacceptable in the practice of paediatric medicine. I do not believe it is possible for us to "feel," to "sense," to "see" for another to this degree. I do not believe it is possible for us to have this kind of particular, highly personal knowledge about another. I have lived with a woman for twenty years and I would not pretend, particularly in her presence, to hazard a guess about such highly individual, highly personal matters. I could only come to know about her feelings, her perspective by her reporting it to me. No one can have this kind of particular knowledge about infants and small children. Infants (literally: "voiceless ones") and children are what we should see and regard as the most morally opaque members of our community. More so than any other members of our community, we cannot know what doing right by them entails or requires of us. We cannot know what they would "feel," "sense" or "see" as right or good for them.

Also, to accept the concept of proxy consent as a legal/ethical right is to confer on parents the power or right to authorize or to refuse to authorize any proposed medical intervention their child might or might not need

(Bartholome, 1979: 271-277). By providing parents this right we would be placing in their hands the power and authority to endanger or neglect their children's medical needs. And, as health care providers, we would have to simply stand by as the health care providers did in response to the parental refusal to give consent to surgical treatment for the infant with Down's syndrome at Johns Hopkins in 1971 and again in Bloomington, Indiana in 1982. Infants and children are more than the products, property, projects or valuable pets of their parents. I have no difficulty in describing the moral standing of children. I see children, just as I see myself, as developing, evolving, (hopefully) growing persons. They are at a slightly earlier phase in the process than I, but I am still learning and I learn a great deal from them! This moral standing as developing persons requires that no one be capable (legally or ethically) of treating them as products, property, projects or pets.

It is also important to remember that children's health care providers, such as paediatricians, by virtue of their social roles and relationships with their child-patients have legal and ethical duties and obligations which exist independently of any parental wishes, desires, and/or "consentings." The social roles played by child health professionals have attached to them specific duties that are owed to their patients, in this case to their child-patients. In addition, when a health care professional enters into a relationship with a particular infant or child, an interpersonal relationship is established. In the law the relationship is characterized as a "fiduciary" relationship. On the basis of the existence of such a relationship many arguments can be launched about particular moral and legal obligations owed to the individual children involved (Robertson and Fost, 1976). For example, one of the most important ethical (and legal) obligations involved is that once such a relationship is established the provider may not abandon the child. If the child's parents do not want a particular provider to continue to provide care to their child, the provider may terminate the relationship after he/she has identified a provider who is willing to accept the responsibility of providing care to the child. The health care professional is a moral agent who has a fiduciary "contract" with the child-patient or, if you prefer, is involved in a "covenant" relationship with the child.

If we are willing to reject the concept of "proxy consent" where does this leave us? Such a rejection allows us to see the more morally appropriate way of talking about such decisions. Given these serious limitations of the concept of proxy consent, decision-making involving the health care of infants and children should be based on the concept of a shared responsibility to respond to the imperiled child; on a shared responsibility to protect the health, welfare and interests of the child. The parents should have a voice. I would argue that what might best be called "informed parental permission" should always be sought prior to any medical intervention or decision to withhold or withdraw. Obviously, this requirement would not be required in the case of an emergency. However, such parental permission should not be treated as a sufficient basis in and of itself to justify either intervention or a decision to withhold/withdraw. And, parental refusal to give permission to an intervention or to a proposal to withhold/withdraw does not relieve the provider of duties or obligations he/she might have to the infant/child.

The Role of the Child and the Concept of Assent

Given the above description of the proper role of the parents in decision-making, what of the role of the child? One of the most serious impediments to any discussion of the role of the child is that, under the influence of our legal system, we have come to think of concepts such as competency or capacity for decision-making and the like as what might be called "threshold" concepts (Gaylin, 1982: 27-57). One is incompetent until he/she has passed a particular threshold point, like attaining a particular age. We have also come to think about such concepts as either present or absent. Often judges or others are asked to declare whether a particular person is or is not competent, for example. We should not allow our thinking about such concepts to be dictated by the requirements of concepts in law. The reality is that competence or capacity are developments and that we are all more or less competent depending on the particular tasks at hand, i.e., that competence and capacity are relative. Children should be decision-making persons with developing capacities to participate in decision making not only about what food to eat, or what clothes to wear, or how to style hair and hundreds of other decisions; but, also, as having an evolving capacity to participate in decisions about their health and their health care. We have learned this lesson primarily from children with chronic illnesses. We have discovered that it is essential that they see themselves as involved in decision-making; as having some control over what happens to them. We have discovered that in many situations they know their disease (through their ongoing experience with the "illness" it causes) better than anyone else. We have discovered that frequently they can do a better job of taking care of their disease than any other caretaker. So our ethical obligation is to involve children to the extent of their capacity for sharing in decision-making rather than attempting to make judgments about which children have reached or achieved this magical thing called competence. We should assume that the child has an evolving capacity for competence and involve him/her to the extent that is possible.

I would like to argue that as the paediatric patient develops he or she gradually displaces his/her parents as the primary guardian of personal health and as the primary partner in decision-making about health care. The verb "displaces" is extremely important in that sentence. I worked on the study of that verb for several years! The idea is that in the partnership arrangement that should characterize medical decision-making, the parents get pushed out of the picture by the developing child. An important task of the paediatric provider is to facilitate this process. When it is appropriate we need to be ready to say: "Excuse me, I need to talk to your daughter alone. Would you please wait out in the waiting room." Or: "Next time John comes in for his appointment, would you mind just dropping him off and coming back for him later. I need to work on strengthening my relationship with your son." Or, even more importantly, "I'm going to perform a pelvic examination on your daughter now, Mr. Brown. I think she and I would both be more comfortable if you were not in the room. Thanks."

Moving from this "every-day" context to that of the withholding/withdrawal of life-sustaining treatment raises additional problems about the role of the child in this process. One of the biggest hurdles is that a deliberate decision to forego in this context involves, in an important sense, a child "facing" his/her own death. That is, if a child is to participate in such a decision, he/she would be doing so recognizing that such a decision was a decision in which his/her death was at stake. For many adults, the idea of children making choices in the face of their own deaths is almost unthinkable. In our relationships with children we have powerful needs to see them as needing our protection. We need to see ourselves as playing an important role in taking care of them, in shielding them from the harshness of "the real world." Most of us have a hard enough time talking to them about sex, much less death!

I would argue that most of our apprehension when confronted by such an idea rests on the projection of our own fears and problems onto our children. In fact, we are now in the position to know that like many other aspects of "their reality," children have conceptions of death and dying that are radically different from our own (Raimbault, 1981). It is terribly important for health care providers to keep the "problems" separate. As health care providers we will be faced with our own set of challenges and problems in working with a dying child. We will also be faced with the difficult task of helping parents deal with their problems with their child dying. The parents will have their own set of problems. And, most importantly, the child will have a set of challenges and problems to deal with as he/she faces his/her own death. It is essential that we work on our resistance to the idea of letting children "own" problems like these. For example, in paediatric oncology there was a long tradition of deceiving children and engaging in elaborate conspiracies with parents to conceal from children the reality of their diseases (Leiken, 1983: 61-71). One would like to think that this practice came to an end because health care professionals realized that it was wrong to lie to children, to deceive them, to deprive them of the truth. However, the practice came to an end primarily because it was discovered that the children knew what was going on; that they frequently felt angry and cheated; and that they reluctantly joined into the conspiracy because they took it as what they were supposed to do and in order to protect their parents!

How should we go about characterizing an appropriate role for the child? We should consider a concept such as that of child assent to delineate this role. What does it mean to "assent"? I would argue that "assent" includes at least three basic ingredients or "elements," if you prefer that term.

The first is the duty of the health care professional to assist the child in developing an age-appropriate (developmentally) awareness of the nature of his/her illness. Basically, this duty requires that the professional help the child to become aware, to come to understand, to come to know what is going on in terms of their health and life. Although it would be too long an aside, please note the world of difference between such a duty and the "broadcasting" of information to (at) the child. As professionals we are just beginning to become aware of the demands of "real" communication, of a genuine "dialogue" with our patients.

The second element is the duty of the professional to disclose the nature of the proposed intervention or, in our case, the proposed withholding/withdrawal. Particularly in the case of children such a disclosure requirement should focus primarily on what the child is likely to experience rather than merely on what will (or will not) be done.

The third element is an obligation to see the child's expression of willingness to undergo the proposed treatment or to its being withheld/withdrawn. And to hear (and respect as much as possible) the child's dissent or expression of unwillingness. Obviously, this is crucial. To withhold or withdraw a life-sustaining treatment from a child without their expressed willingness that this be done or in the face of their expressed opposition to such a decision would be at least *prima facie* unethical.

The Role of the Health Care Professional

Given these descriptions of the role of both parents and children in such decisions, I would like to turn to a brief description of what is the appropriate role of the health care professional. I am not arguing that this is a definitive and comprehensive analysis of this role, but rather a way of describing this important set of tasks. I have listed what might be called six ethical characteristics or aspects of this role. First, as I argued in the section on parents, health care professionals have legal and ethical duties and obligations which are owed to the child-patient. A definitive listing of all these duties and obligations is beyond the scope of this presentation. As examples, such a list would include the duty of physicians and nurses to be competent and to render competent medical and nursing care to the child;

the obligation to "do no harm"; the duty not to abandon a child in peril; the obligation to tell the truth; and others.

A second aspect is the duty of the provider to determine and to define the nature of the child's condition, his/her disease(s) and associated problems; and, to provide the parents and the child (to the extent of his/her capacity for understanding) an accurate prognosis or description of the "natural history" of these disease(s)/problems. This is a step often neglected by providers. Basically, it is the story of what is likely to happen if the provider does not intervene. It is essential that the parents/child be given a picture of this likely course of events since professionals have an almost irresistible tendency to overestimate our power to intervene in these processes. Much of the "power of modern scientific medicine" is the power to have some influence, to have some degree of impact, to modify the disease process, but not to "fix it," to "make the problem go away," to cure, to restore to health, to "heal." Such candor about the limitations of our power is an essential, and neglected, aspect of a genuine dialogue.

The third aspect of the professional's role is to define with the parent and child the range and nature of possible or feasible responses to these disease(s) problems or the "treatment options." In the context of this particular topic, it is essential that this definitional process include explicit discussion of those options that are futile or largely useless in terms of benefits to the child. In terms of narrowing the range of possible options it is sometimes helpful to start at the "edges" by analysis of the "natural history" (what is likely to happen if we do nothing); and then delineation of those possible options that are unlikely to be beneficial in terms of the interests of the child.

The fourth aspect of the professional's role is to delineate the likely consequences of those alternative courses of action which are likely to be of at least some benefit, especially in terms of the "costs" of such alternatives in addition to any anticipated benefits. I use the word "costs" in the broad sense of a comprehensive assessment of the burdens that the treatment will or may impose on the child and the family. I do not mean to rule out consideration of the economic factors, but they are only one of many "costs" that need to be considered. In order to compensate for our built-in tendency to focus on potential benefits, a delineation is required that gives priority to a consideration of costs or burdens; and, that such a priority or lexical ordering is in keeping with the importance afforded the duty to "above all do no harm" in traditional professional ethics.

The fifth aspect of the role is what I would call acceptance of the responsibility of assisting the child and parents in selecting "the right" course of action. Obviously, there is no absolute or ultimately right course of action (at least that we can know about as mere mortals). "The right" in this context can be understood to mean things like: "what appears to us to be the least wrong" or "what seems to be the best course of action under these circumstances" or others. Basically, my argument is that the health care professional's job is not to dump a mountain of information and "treatment options" on the table and then stand back and "let them decide." Our job is not merely that of providing people with information. Our task includes an honest sharing with our patients of our perspective, our feelings, our thoughts and our judgments. In our effort to avoid the paternalism of making judgments for our patients and their families, we must remember our obligation to make judgments with our patients and their families rather than abdicating this responsibility in the name of respect for autonomy or the rights of patients. Patients, particularly children, have a "right" to a health care provider who is a moral agent, who is involved with them in the process and responsibility of decision-making.

The last aspect of this role which I would ask you to examine is the set of actions undertaken by the professional to implement the course of action selected. And, I would add, to do so not only competently, but with compassion and caring. In the context of our topic, we are discussing a course of action that involves withholding or withdrawing life-sustaining treatment. One of the most vocal and recurring complaints against providers in the context of such decisions is that patients often hear and experience such decisions as involving abandonment. It is important to see that in making such decisions we are *not* making a decision to stop providing medical or nursing care. It is to decide not to use a particular treatment modality. If the family of a child with refractory metastatic cancer is told: "We've done all we can do for your son; medicine has nothing left to offer him," you can bet money that they will end up in Tijuana, Mexico or in the hands of some charlatan. He and his parents will hear (and likely experience) abandonment. On the other hand, if after appropriate discussion of what has and is going on with this boy the parents were told: "We're going to continue to provide the best care we can for your son; to provide him everything we can to help make his life as comfortable and full as possible; and, we do not think we should give him more anticancer drugs because they don't seem to be doing anything other than making him feel more sick"; that will not be heard as "we're going to stop chemotherapy" and (unstated) "abandon your son." The decision to withhold or to withdraw a particular life-sustaining treatment will always be a decision to begin to provide another (and perhaps more demanding and difficult!) mode of care. In my experience, "only caring" is frequently more time-consuming, more psychologically demanding, and requires more "hands-on" care than decisions to use or to continue a piece of life-sustaining technology.

Criteria for Decisions to Withhold/Withdraw

To this point I have attempted a description of the appropriate role of parents, the child-patient and the professional providers in making decisions to withhold/withdraw life-sustaining treatment. I would now like to turn to examination of the question of what criteria should these individuals use in consideration of such decisions? One way of understanding this would be to say that up to this point we have addressed the "Who?" question and described in considerable detail the complex ways in which these individuals might go about sharing in the process and responsibility for making decisions. We now turn to a "What?" question: what criteria ought to be used? I have listed and will briefly discuss eight criteria that have been proposed for use in this context. As you will see there is considerable overlap between some of them and there may well be other candidates that I have left out of this brief analysis. My analysis of these candidates will conclude with an argument that none of them are sufficient as substantive criteria. The use of these criteria may (and more likely may not) be helpful in an effort to understand the ethical aspects of these decisions. But none of them is adequate; and the lack of any clear, accepted criteria for such decisions demands that we examine other, very different approaches to these problems.

1. *Do whatever "can" be done.*

Another way of stating this criterion is: do that which is "medically feasible." Use of such a criterion would virtually rule out a decision to withhold or withdraw since any such decision is a decision to not do something that could be done. This approach also forces infants and children to die "up against the wall" of everything that modern medicine can do. It is not as hard on physicians as it is on the nursing care professionals who have to implement it. It is terribly hard on families. I would argue it is such a burden on infants and children that it can properly be called "torture." Although I do not have a lot of respect for much of the work he has done in this area, Raymond Duff from Yale-New Haven Medical Center came up with a powerful metaphor for such a policy: "Medical Vietnam" (Duff, 1981). As a graduate of the 60's, I can feel the power of this metaphor.

2. *Do whatever prolongs life.*

Alternatively, "preserve life." One of the most peculiar aspects of medical ethics as it evolved in the United States during the nineteenth and early twentieth centuries (and I am not sure how much of it carried over into Canada), is that health care professionals of this era began conceiving of themselves as having a duty to prolong life. The source of this self-imposed duty is not at all clear even to the best medical historians of the period (Amundsen, 1978). However, use of this criterion, particularly in the new age of technological medicine, has the perverse effect of demanding that aggressive treatment be provided until there is no evidence or signs of life. The philosophical roots of this approach lie in something called vitalism. One very severe deficiency in the criterion is that it would deny to our patients the status "dying." It denies the existence of a category of interventions that might prolong life but be cruel, excessively burdensome and/or "only prolong dying."

3. *Do that which is "medically indicated."*

Often this criterion is expressed as the result of the exercise of something called "reasonable medical judgment." In the context of this discussion, for example, the United States Congress recently passed what is called the Child Abuse and Neglect Amendments of 1984 in which the federal legislature defined what it termed "medical neglect" (Child Abuse Amendments, 1984). Medical neglect was defined as the failure to provide "medically indicated treatment" to an infant suffering from a life-threatening medical condition. "Medically indicated treatment" was defined as the treatment that was felt to be indicated in the "reasonable medical judgement" of a physician. One critical assumption made by the legislators was that these terms referred to some objective body of knowledge; something that some have called medical science or the science of medicine. I would argue that the phrase "medically indicated" as it has been used historically hides the moral or ethical dimensions of medicine practice. Medicine, nursing and all the health care professions are in their practice moral, not technical enterprises. Therefore, there is no such thing as a course of action that is indicated by the science of medicine. Every decision made by a practicing health care professional that has influence on the health, welfare or life of a patient is a moral or ethical decision. Clearly all such decisions should involve and be informed by the knowledge and technology of medical (or nursing) science, but so-called medical science only tells us what can be done, not what ought to be done. Thus, strictly speaking, this criterion fails since there can be no such thing as a "medically indicated" course of action which involves care of patients.

4. *Do not prolong dying.*

This criterion was also incorporated into the Child Abuse and Neglect Amendments of 1984 as an "exception" to the rule requiring "medically indicated" treatment. Again, a crucial assumption was made by the legislators; namely, that the word "dying" referred to a clinical condition that could be defined in some objective terms. We have yet to come up with a definition of the word dying that can be operationalized in a clinical setting. It has been assumed that doctors and/or nurses simply knew or could tell when a patient is dying. It is almost as if many conceive of there being some test or series of tests; that a blood sample could be sent to the lab and the lab slip would come back stamped "dying." The problem is, dying is not a medical diagnosis. It is not a medical syndrome or even a medical condition. If it can be labelled at all, it is more like an existential state like "living" or, perhaps, a kind of living. But philosophers have been struggling for all of recorded history to come up with a definition for "living." So, the problem is that although it sounds like an appealing criterion, when you take it into the clinical setting things get very sticky. When you stand at the foot of the bed and ask: "Is this patient dying?", How do you know? What kind of question is this? Who can tell?

Although I think this criterion points to an area that deserves study and may yield some helpful hints to those facing these decisions, it is not a criterion that is of much help to us now.

5. *Quality of life.*

Often this consideration is used as a proposed corrective to the "sanctity of life" position or as a check on the vitalism of "prolong/preserve life." Quality-of-life language snuck into the thinking about medicine and health care in the 1950's. A great deal of critical work has been done on the concept and the "ideologies" of those who have used it (Edlund and Tancredi, 1985). I do not think it can carry much ethical weight since it is primarily a very ambiguous and confusing slogan. It reminds me of what Saul Alinsky used to say about ethics (Alinsky, 1971). Alinsky was very aware that anyone who wanted to induce change, to launch a viable social movement, needed to sugar coat anything they called for or did in the language of ethics. It is important to understand at least one very serious ambiguity in this concept. The ambiguity resides in the word "life." In English, unlike many other languages, we have only this one noun which we use to refer to some radically different aspects of what is meant by "life." For example, most of us regard talk of "quality of life" as a kind of reforming influence in health care. It calls attention to the idea that physicians should be concerned with more than pathophysiology, more than the discovery and description of diseases; that we should attend to the experience of the patient, the lived-life of the patient. We are asked to attend to the "illness", i.e., the patient's experience of what it is like to live with his/her disease(s); and, to be concerned with the "quality" of life. In this context the word "life" is used to refer to an individual's experiences; life in the autobiographical sense; life as lived or experienced.

However, this same word "life" has a very different meaning and when incorporated into the concept "quality of life" is not only not reforming, but dangerous. We also use this noun in a biographical sense. We use it to refer to the duration of time an individual spends on this planet; to describe what he/she did or did not do. In this sense use of the concept invites health care professions to make judgments about the "quality" or lack of "quality" of others' lives; invites professionals to provide treatment to a patient on the basis of judgments made by the professionals about the life of that individual. As a matter of fact, if one looks at what was regarded at the time as the finest medical profession in the world, namely that of Germany in the early decades of this century, it was precisely this concept that unleashed a widespread slaughter of not Jews or Poles or Slavs, but of German citizens (LaChat, 1975). Tens of thousands of German men, women and children were not only denied medical care, but killed on the basis of their lack of an adequate "quality of life." We even incorporated one of this profession's key concepts into our contemporary debate about newborns with a variety of severe problems when we talked of "defectives" and "defective newborns."

Although in its autobiographical sense we can use the concept of "quality of life" in our work with older children and adolescents who can report to us their perceived or experienced quality of life, it has very limited utility in decisions involving infants and young children. And, given the dangers inherent in the use of the concept in the biographical sense, it has limited value as a substantive criterion.

6. *Do that which would be approved by a "reasonable person."*

In the legal context this is often referred to as the "reasonable man" standard. Although there is something appealing about the idea that decisions in order to be ethical should be based on "good reasons" or that "reason" should prevail, there are serious questions about how to go about putting such a criterion into practice. My favourite example, returning to the "Hopkins Case," was provided by the paediatric surgeon in that case. He shared with me that the way he made such decisions was to imagine himself in the situation of the infant and then decide what to do. As he was describing this exercise in imagination, I had this perverse image in my mind of him floating through the air into the infant's isolette. His adult body was packed into the clear plastic box filling it so completely that the baby was squirted out through one of the portholes in the back of the isolette onto the floor. He regarded this as empathy; as application of reason and the Golden Rule. I saw it as a sincere, but misguided exercise. We cannot place ourselves in other people's shoes. In fact, genuine empathy demands that we actually imagine what it is like for this particular individual to be in his/her own shoes! How does one apply reasonableness to the situation of a handicapped newborn? Is it reasonable to want to receive life-sustaining treatment if the life one is likely to experience will be lived in a wheelchair? Will be marked by mental retardation? Who knows?

7. Do that which the parents/surrogates select.

Even if one rejects the concept of proxy consent as I have suggested, an argument can be made that the course of action preferred or selected by the parents should be given priority. Since no one can know what the infant or child would have us do; and, since there are no good criteria for making these decisions, why not give the benefit of the doubt to the parents. "After all," it is argued, "it's their child." Often the rationale given is that health care providers are poorly trained to make these complex "value judgments" and/or health care providers should not "impose their values" on the family. I think the temptation to dump this "hot potato" onto the parents is one that we must resist. The use of the possessive pronouns "their," "my" and the like in descriptors such as "their child" or "my son" is ambiguous (Langham, 1979). On one view such words are used merely to denote status in a relationship, e.g., to designate paternity. In another more common and dangerous sense they are used to designate ownership, as in "my car," "my house" and "my son." As health care professionals we also must resist the temptation to abdicate our moral responsibility to our patient. It is in those cases which are most complex, most uncertain, most perplexing that they most need our involvement and advocacy.

8. *Do what is in the child's best interests.*

Of all the criteria that have been proposed I am most comfortable with this "child-oriented/focused" one. However, it does not and, I believe, cannot function as a substantive criterion. At most it tells us to attend to the child as we make decisions. The metaphor I use to describe how it works is that of the directional beacon in the fog. In the fog of ignorance, uncertainty, ambiguity and perplexity that permeates decision-making about infants and children, this beacon serves to keep the party of responsible adults focused; seeking to do that which might be in the child's best interests. It also functions in a negative sense by limiting the extent to which other factors and other loyalties should be allowed to enter into the dialogue, e.g., the interests of the family, of the society and the like (Macklin, 1982: 265-301).

Procedure, Procedural Justice and "Due Process"

Given the absence of any satisfactory substantive criteria we ought to try a different approach to this aspect of the problem. The question that I would ask you to consider might be called the "How?" question. The idea is that we ought to do our best to insure that withholding and withdrawal decisions are made well; with appropriate deliberateness and caution; with "due process." Instead of the seemingly non-productive search for better, more directive substantive criteria, we should focus, at least in part, on procedure. Ask yourself: "What would a procedural mechanism look like that would do justice to what is at stake in these decisions?"

I would like to describe one such procedure. First, I would ask that all parties to the procedure agree to the utilization of the "best interest of the child" focus. That is to say that the primary loyalty or the highest priority of the people involved in the procedure would be determined as the interests of the child whose life is "on the line." Secondly, we would stipulate that the decision be one in which what I am calling the primary decision-makers share in the responsibility and reach a consensus. Obviously, how one defines the circle of primary decision-makers is critical. I would argue that any such circle would need to include the child-patient (to the extent of his/her capacity to participate), the parents and key health care providers. I use that language rather than "the doctor" for a number of reasons. I think we need to be much more honest about who it is that is providing care to hospitalized infants and children. The primary providers to this population of children are nurses. To make a decision to withhold or withdraw life-sustaining treatment from a patient and to fail to involve the individual who is most intimately involved in that patient's care makes no sense. In many situations involving infants the nurse is the only source of what might be called particular knowledge, i.e., the knowledge of how this particular infant is experiencing and responding to attempts to provide care. So, that would give us the patient, the parents, the primary care nurse(s), the attending physician and other physicians as necessary. For example, if the treatment being contemplated involves a surgical procedure, it would seem that the paediatric surgeon ought to be a part of this circle. And arguments can be made to include others on the basis of some special status. For example, a grandparent may be a primary caretaker. Or a child may have been a patient of a particular therapist for five years.

A third feature of the procedure is a back-up system for situations in which the members of the primary circle are unable to reach consensus; or in which there is persistent perplexity about the ethical issues at stake; or, in which a member of the primary circle wants the back-up system to provide review of the decision that has been reached. This is where the idea of establishing hospital-based review mechanisms comes in. In the States the majority of large tertiary hospitals have established ethics committees as this mechanism (Ross, 1986). The idea is to set in place a procedural mechanism that would be available to the parties involved in these difficult decisions to allow a genuine dialogue to take place; to allow disagreements to be aired and settled; and to allow decisions to be made to withhold or withdraw life-sustaining treatment without involvement of the legal system. The argument is that taking these difficult ethical decisions away from the bedside, out of the hospital community and into the arena of the courtroom can seriously distort the issues. Making them legal decisions, taking them into court, tears them out of the reality, the context, in which they arise. The argument in favour of such review is based on the idea that the committee can provide a diversity of perspectives brought by its members and represents an impartial, disinterested yet informed group made up of individuals who are members of

38

the same hospital community. Such a review requirement is also an indication of the awareness that such decisions do have as an important and fundamental aspect depriving a child of his/her life.

Summary

Decisions to withhold/withdraw life-sustaining treatment are ethical decisions that involve deliberately depriving children of their lives (thus demanding meticulous attention and care), and, decisions to allow a child to die (thus demanding strength and courage). Informed parental permission (and not "proxy consent") is an ethical (and legal) requirement in such decisions. Parents must share in the responsibility to make these decisions with both their child and child's health care providers. The child-patient should be empowered to participate to the extent of his/her capacity; and the solicitation of his/her assent is an ethical requirement. The role of the health care provider includes: meticulous diagnosis and prognosis; disclosure and dialogue regarding the treatment options; an active sharing in the decision-making; and, the provision of continuing care even when a decision has been made to withhold/withdraw some particular treatment. Given the absence of any clear substantive criteria for making such decisions, a circle of primary decision-makers (with a primary commitment to the pursuit of the best interest of the child) should share in the responsibility for making such decisions with the "back-up system" of formal review by a hospital ethics committee or similar mechanism.

REFERENCES

Alinsky, S. 1971. *Rules for Radicals.* New York: Vintage Books.

Amundsen, D. 1978. The physician's obligation to prolong life: A medical duty without classical roots. *Hastings Center Report* 8: 23-31.

Bartholome, W. G. 1979. The child patient: Do parents have the right to decide? *The Law-Medicine Relation: A Philosophical Critique,* edited by S. Spicker. Boston: D. Reidel.

Bartholome, W. G. 1982. Proxy consent in the medical context: The infant as person. *Philosophy, Children and the Family: #1 Child Nurturance,* Vol. I, edited by A. C. Cafagna. New York: Plenum Press: 335-351.

Child Abuse Amendments of 1984, PUB. L. No. 98 - 457, tit. 1, secs. 121-128, 98 STAT. 1749 (Codified at 42 U.S.C. 5101-5103. (Supp 1985)).

Duff, R. S. 1981. Counselling families and deciding care in severely defective children: A way of coping with 'Medical Vietnam.' *Paediatrics* 67: 315-320.

Edlund, M. and L. R. Tancredi. 1985. Quality of Life: An ideological critique. *Perspectives in Biology and Medicine* 28 (4): 591-607.

Engelhardt, Jr., H. T. 1986. *The Foundations of Bioethics.* New York: Oxford University Press.

Faden, R. R. and T. L. Beauchamp. 1986. *A History and Theory of Informed Consent.* New York: Oxford University Press.

Gaylin, W. 1982. Competence: No longer all or none. *Who Speaks for the Child: The Problems of Proxy Consent,* edited by W. Gaylin and R. Macklin. New York: Plenum Press.

Katz, J. 1984. *The Silent World of Doctor and Patient.* New York: Free Press.

Kennedy Foundation. 1971. Who Shall Survive (Film). Washington, D. C.: Joseph P. Kennedy, Jr. Foundation.

Kubler-Ross, E. 1975. *Death: The Final Stage of Growth.* Englewood Cliffs, N. J.: Prentice-Hall.

LaChat, M. 1975. Utilitarian reasoning in Nazi medical policy: Some preliminary investigations. *Linacre Quarterly* (Feb.): 14-37.

Langham, P. 1979. Parental consent: Its justification and limitations. *Clinical Research* 27: 1-18.

Leiken, S. 1983. An ethical issue in paediatric cancer care: Non-disclosure of a fatal diagnosis. *Ethical Issues in the Treatment of Children and Adolescents,* edited by J. Silber. Thorafare, N. J.: Slack, Inc.

40

Macklin, R. 1982. Return to the best interest of the child. *Who Speaks for the Child: The Problems of Proxy Consent,* edited by W. Gaylin and R. Macklin. New York: Plenum Press.

Melden, A. I. 1980. Do infants have moral rights? *Whose Child?: Children's Rights, Parental Authority and State Power,* edited by W. Aiken and M. LaFollette. New Jersey: Rowman and Littlefield: 199-221.

Murray, T. H. and A. L. Caplan (eds.). 1985. *Which Babies Shall Live?: Humanistic Dimensions of the Care of Imperiled Newborns.* Clifton, N. J.: Humana Press.

O'Donovan, O. 1984. *Begotten or Made?* Oxford: Clarendon Press: 49-67.

Raimbault, G. 1981. Children talk about death. *Acta Paediatrica Scandinavica* 70: 179-182.

Ramsey, P. 1970. *The Patient as Person: Explorations in Medical Ethics.* New Haven: Yale University Press.

Robertson, J. A. and N. Fost. 1976. Passive euthanasia of defective newborn infants: Legal considerations. *Journal of Paediatrics* 88: 883-889.

Ross, J. W. 1986. *Handbook for Hospital Ethics Committees.* Chicago: American Hospital Publishing Company.

Veatch, R. M. 1981. *A Theory of Medical Ethics.* New York: Basic Books.

Weir, R. 1984. *Selective Non-treatment of Handicapped Newborns.* New York: Oxford University Press.

Innovative Lifesaving Treatments: Do Children Have A Moral Right To Receive Them?

Terrence F. Ackerman

The human drama which provides the focus for my analysis has become sadly familiar. The parents of a very sick child appeal for help on the television news. Their child needs an innovative, potentially lifesaving treatment, such as a liver transplant. It is very expensive, perhaps more than 100,000 dollars, and they do not have money or insurance coverage. Displays appear in local stores, beckoning us to contribute to the treatment fund. There are raffles, celebrity sports events, car washes and innumerable other fund-raising activities sponsored by churches, youth groups and civic organizations. In some cases, the fund-raising succeeds and the drama shifts to the hospital, perhaps in some distant city, where specialists await those who can make the down payment. In other cases, the physical toll of disease accumulates more swiftly than charitable donations, and the child dies before the down payment is secured.

There are two immediate reactions to these circumstances. One is that parents should not have to beg for money needed to keep their children alive. Although society's resources are limited, we should reserve funds sufficient to provide lifesaving treatments for these children. Failure to guarantee treatment, as a societal commitment, is a morally unconscionable abandonment of those in most dire need. The other reaction is far more cautionary. It is that life is replete with medical misfortunes which wrench at our hearts and perhaps our faith. Nevertheless, society cannot assume responsibility for systematically rectifying the arbitrary hand of fate. Such an undertaking would drain away limited resources for other important societal endeavors, such as education, as well as the funds for other health care programs. It would also necessitate enormous redistribution of wealth that would crush personal freedoms under the weight of state taxation. Rather, we should urge voluntary contributions to charitable funds created to help those in dire medical need.

Both reactions acknowledge that societal resources are limited. But they embody different priorities: one reaction emphasizing the preeminent importance of fulfilling unmet basic health care needs, the other underscoring the costs to other welfare needs and personal freedoms in achieving this goal. These separate reactions anticipate full-blown philosophical positions.

In the 1960's and 1970's, philosophers, theologians and policy analysts argued that persons have a moral right to health care. Only passing attention was devoted to the possibility that serious limits on resources and other pressing social needs might constrain its implementation (Outka, 1976; Veatch, 1976; McCullough, 1979). In the intervening years, the explosion of expensive medical technologies and rapid increases in the costs of government health care programs have forcibly demonstrated that rights to health care cannot be implemented without trading off other important social interests. As a result, even writers who strongly emphasize societal obligations to meet basic welfare needs now carefully avoid the claim that society should fund costly lifesaving treatments, such as liver transplants, for children (Brody, 1981; Daniels, 1985; U. S. President's Commission, 1983; Veatch, 1986).

Indeed, the focal question today is whether it is reasonable to claim a moral right to innovative, but very expensive, lifesaving medical treatments in the face of emerging cost constraints. In this paper, I assess some prominent objects to claim that there is a moral right to receive such treatments at the expense of society. In the next section, I outline the moral framework within which the issue is debated. Subsequently, I evaluate key arguments intended to undercut the view that society has a moral obligation to provide very expensive, lifesaving treatments for its children. The upshot of my analysis is that the claim that children have a moral right to receive these treatments cannot be dismissed as easily as currently thought.

Basic Framework of the Debate

There may be an alternative to rights-based theories as a framework to sort out this ethical issue. One might think in terms of the society as a whole and seek to develop social institutions which recognize the interdependence and the interactions of people rather than concentrating on preserving a sphere of isolation privacy (Sherwin, 1984-1985). Rights language, however, is relatively current with the main opponents of the view that children have a right to expensive, innovative, lifesaving treatments. Ultimately, there are difficulties in settling priority-type conflicts in either approach, but such is the nature of any moral problem.

Unfortunately, many goods are in short supply. Persons with conflicting interests may compete for the possession of these goods. For example, limited government funds allocated to health care may be sought for both sick children seeking liver transplants and retarded children needing developmental services. Similarly, the need for taxation schemes to support these programs may conflict with the interests of other persons in using their income for private purposes. An obligation to provide innovative, lifesaving treatments to paediatric patients at the expense of society must be justified by a theory about how limited goods or services should be distributed. Within moral philosophy, it is the theory of distributive justice which attempts to determine the fair distribution of limited goods or services.

Although there are many differences in rival theories of distributive justice, most recent theories share two important assumptions. These are that persons have an intrinsic worth which they possess just as persons, and that this worth is possessed equally by all persons. An important implication is that whatever society owes persons as a result of their intrinsic worth, it must distribute these goods (such as liberties and welfare goods) in a manner which acknowledges the equal worth of all persons. For example, if the intrinsic worth of persons requires that society provide basic liberties of free speech and movement, then society must assure that persons equally possess them. Commitment to the equal worth of persons does not clarify how to recognize persons as equal when the goods or services being distributed are limited. The principle of equal opportunity is invoked to clarify this matter (Rawls, 1971: 83-90; Daniels, 1985: 36-58; Veatch, 1986: 119-147). The basic idea is that, if each person has intrinsic worth, we should distribute essential social goods in ways which respect equally the opportunity of each to realize his or her life plans or to have a good life. Freedoms to pursue occupational interests, access to educational resources, legal protections and other social goods should be distributed in a manner which shows equal regard for the efforts of persons to implement their life plans.

However, these shared assumptions do not carry us far in deciding whether there is a moral right to receive medical treatment. Even if it is agreed that society must assure that goods distributed through its institutions allow equal opportunity for all persons, the question remains open as to what social goods should be assigned priority. For example, does regard for the worth of persons require that we distribute only liberties such as freedom of movement and speech? Or does it require the distribution of liberties and welfare goods? If it does require the distribution of welfare goods, how should available funds be distributed between health care and other essential welfare goods, such as education, housing and transportation? Within the health care sector itself, how should funds be divided among programs for preventive, acute and rehabilitative services? The attempt to answer these key questions includes evaluating the claim that persons have a moral right to receive very costly, lifesaving medical treatment at the expense of society.

Personal Freedoms and Welfare Goods

Liberties and welfare services are two main categories of goods whose relative importance affects the claim that there is a moral right to medical care. Funding of large-scale welfare programs requires that governments redistribute funds from the wealthier members of society to cover the costs of these programs. Redistributive mechanisms (e.g., taxation) by their very nature reduce the freedom of the comparatively well-off members of society to retain and use their wealth for private purposes. As a result, if we place high priority upon the distribution of liberties, then there is little basis for the claim that persons have a moral right to receive innovative, but very expensive lifesaving medical treatments. Redistributive mechanisms used to generate funds to support such a right would undermine the freedoms assigned a higher moral priority.

This kind of position is illustrated by Tristram Engelhardt, Jr.'s view of distributive justice. Engelhardt argues that persons gain ownership of things when they refashion, remold or mingle their labor with such objects not already similarly owned by someone else (Engelhardt, 1986: 130). Persons may freely sell or otherwise transfer rights of ownership to other persons, and they may also justly acquire rights of ownership to additional objects through the same process. However, once ownership is established, persons have a fundamental right not to be interfered with in the possession of objects. These rights of ownership include justly acquired monetary resources. The distribution of welfare goods among the members of society is just only if these fundamental rights of ownership and transfer are not violated.

Engelhardt does not completely reject welfare programs which use redistributed monies to fund expensive lifesaving treatments. However, he would insist that these programs rely on voluntary contributions of money from members of the community. Persons are free to contribute their money, but there is no obligation to provide assistance to children in need. Since there is no obligation, children have no moral right to receive innovative and costly lifesaving treatment at the expense of society. At best, access to these treatments might be available for some children, but only if there is sufficient charitable giving of the sort currently sought by families without adequate resources to cover catastrophic health care expenses.

However, there are serious weaknesses in Engelhardt's position. The basic assumptions underlying recent views regarding distributive justice are that persons have intrinsic worth just as persons, and that all persons equally possess this worth. Engelhardt narrowly interprets respect for the intrinsic worth of persons to mean that we should equally respect the capacity of persons to direct their own lives. Our responsibilities to assure equal opportunity would be fulfilled by protecting liberties persons need to autonomously implement their life plans. Since personal resources are important for persons to implement their life plans, recognition of ownership rights is essential.

This narrow interpretation of intrinsic worth seems seriously incomplete. Persons have another distinctive capacity – the capacity for acute suffering. If this is also a preeminent capacity of persons, why should it always be trumped by respect for the capacity of other persons for autonomous self-direction? Suppose we allow children with treatable life-threatening conditions to die because their families are unable to pay for the costs of treatment, while simultaneously refusing to secure the necessary funds from the extravagantly rich. Have these children been shown equal regard for their intrinsic worth? If the answer is "no," then Engelhardt is incorrect that respect for personal freedom should always outweigh the concern to remove harms which threaten the lives of other persons.

The same basic problem can be approached from another perspective. If the capacity for self-direction is what makes persons deserving of our respect, then regard for *any* needs of their personal freedoms should always outweigh the restrictions imposed by redistributive schemes designed to fulfill *any* needs of other persons. However, it seems clear that personal freedoms vary in their degree of moral importance. Freedom of speech, physical movement, religious belief and bodily security seem obviously more central to respect for the worth of persons than the freedom to purchase twenty-eight expensive sports cars for their private collection.

Similarly, the needs of persons differ in the degree to which guarantee of their fulfillment is central to our expression of respect. For example, meeting the needs of persons for adequate health care is surely more important to recognition of their intrinsic worth than meeting their needs to take extended summer vacations at the beach. This is the intuition underlying attempts to define certain basic or essential needs.

In attempting to show respect for all persons in circumstances where their respective interests conflict, the specific type of liberties denied and the needs fulfilled must be weighed. A scale of moral importance will give greater weight to liberties or needs which are most basic to recognition of their intrinsic moral worth. Specifically, basic needs will possess greater moral importance than tangential personal liberties. Conversely, basic personal liberties will possess greater moral weight than tangential personal needs.

Thus, the fact that redistributive schemes restrict some personal freedoms does not necessarily show that they are unjust. If there is abundant wealth in the possession of private individuals which might be used to meet the unfulfilled basic needs of others, and their redistribution does not violate basic liberties, then these resources should be redistributed on a compulsory basis to meet unfulfilled basic needs. If these resources are not redistributed, then we fail to show respect for persons as beings who have a distinct capacity for acute physical and emotional suffering. Engelhardt's argument against the compulsory redistribution of funds needed to support a right to expensive, lifesaving treatments for children does not succeed.

Health Care and Other Welfare Goods

Even if concerns about restricting personal freedoms do not override the claim that children have a right to receive innovative lifesaving treatment at the expense of society, additional obstacles remain in establishing that right. Once we admit a societal obligation to provide for the basic needs of its members as an affirmation of their personal worth, new problems of distributive justice arise. There are many basic or essential needs besides the need for health care. They include needs for housing, clothing, food, education and preservation of physical security. The ability of persons to meet these basic needs through their own efforts may vary greatly. Moreover, different persons will require greater assistance in meeting some of these needs (say, the need for health care) than in meeting other needs (say, the need for adequate housing). Thus the interest of persons in different patterns of distribution of limited resources among basic needs may seriously conflict.

The equal opportunity principle also provides a principled way to set priorities among competing basic needs. Its application to the distribution of welfare goods involves two components. First, it assigns priority in funding decisions to welfare goods which have a comparatively greater bearing than others on the opportunity of persons to implement their life plans. Second, since some persons lack more of essential goods than other persons through no fault of their own, the principle requires that less advantaged persons receive more of society's resources in order to provide them with the opportunity for a good life comparable to the opportunity of other persons. Using these two guidelines, priorities can be set for the distribution of basic welfare goods.

However, theorists who invoke the equal opportunity principle usually avoid the conclusion that needs for expensive lifesaving therapy are likely to achieve funding priority (Daniels, 1981: 173). Norman Daniels claims that deciding what resources to use and what needs to meet "require careful moral judgment and a wealth of empirical knowledge about the effects of alternative allocation" on equal opportunity (Daniels, 1985: 54). If supplying a certain service to everyone who needs one would do more to ensure equality of opportunity than providing catastrophic health care, then a distribution program for the service would have funding priority (Daniels, 1981: 171-172).

Similarly, despite his commitment to the equal opportunity approach, Robert Veatch is extremely cautious in his claims about how much of its redistributed resources society should devote to health care expenditures. For example, Veatch asks how much of society's resources persons would be willing to devote to the needs of the mentally retarded if they were placed in the hypothetical situation of not knowing that they themselves would be mentally retarded (Dworkin, 1981). While he argues that persons would be willing to spend more than is now devoted to the needs of the retarded, he is uncertain what the upper limit of funding would be (Veatch, 1986: 158). He must draw a similar conclusion about fatal diseases requiring innovative, but very expensive lifesaving treatment. If we cannot be sure that persons in the hypothetical situation would consider an appropriate upper limit on expenditures for treatment of life-threatening disease, then there is no firm basis for asserting a socially guaranteed right to receive innovative, but very expensive therapy.

The crucial issue is whether the equal opportunity principle provides any basis for asserting that catastrophic health care needs should receive high priority in the allocation of limited funds among health care and other welfare needs. Although Daniels and Veatch cannot find such theoretical grounds, a firm basis for this priority can be established within the framework of the equal opportunity principle. The key point is that the occurrence of life-threatening illness constitutes the most extreme threat to the opportunity for a good life. While this claim may be true for all persons (Ost, 1987), there are various ways by which one can build a stronger case for children. For example, the children have yet to live their lives, more so than adults, and have not participated in lifestyles leading to their health problems nor in the political process informing allocation decisions (Bartholome, 1987). Seriously ill children have no opportunity to implement life plans when considered *vis-à-vis* their healthy counterparts if they succumb to their disease. Equalization of opportunity for children requires the provision of those welfare goods (i.e., catastrophic health care) which protect the most basic precondition for implementation of their life plans – life itself. Thus, if equality of opportunity is the goal of distributive policies, there is a strong theoretical basis for placing high priority on fulfillment of serious medical needs as compared to other welfare needs.

This point is often overlooked because of the failure to distinguish between the goal of maximizing opportunity among members of society and the goal of equalizing opportunity. Maximization of opportunity concerns maximal *average* improvement in the ability of members of society to implement their life plans. If optimal average improvement in opportunity is the basis of funding allocation decisions, then other welfare goods may assume much higher funding priority than health care. For example, setting the highest priority on the educational needs of society's members may result in a tremendous explosion of industrial and technical productivity. The resulting economic surge may result in maximal average improvement in opportunity for the members of society. By contrast, sinking funds into the health care needs of society's medically worse-off members may constitute a drain on resources otherwise available for economic growth. Nevertheless, if we take seriously the notion of equal intrinsic worth as the basis of just distribution, then our goal in setting funding priorities is the equalization, not the maximization, of opportunity.

It might be contended that this line of reasoning leads to unacceptable consequences for resource allocation. If implementation of the equal opportunity principle requires sinking resources into the worse-off cases, and the worse-off members of society are persons whose lives are threatened by illness, then little of society's resources will be available for meeting other basic needs of its members. However, two considerations deflect this concern. First, there are other unfulfilled basic needs which threaten the lives of children. These include inadequate food, housing and physical security. Even accepting the above implication of the equal opportunity principle, attention to these other basic needs will demand high priority for the same reason as catastrophic health care – failure to fulfill these needs endangers the lives, and consequently the opportunity, of children who are unable to fulfill these needs through no fault of their own. Second, the ability of society to address these various life-threatening needs affecting its worse-off members depends on investment in developing other key welfare goods, such as educational resources. Failure to develop these other goods ultimately stunts the effectiveness and efficiency with which life-threatening needs can be met. For example, the development of medical treatment is dependent upon a good educational system. Development of other welfare goods such as education simultaneously enriches the opportunities of less-disadvantaged persons to achieve their life plans (e.g., through education and research).

Thus, once we accept the equal opportunity principle as a basis for allocating funds among various categories of welfare needs, there are good reasons for asserting that catastrophic health care should receive high funding priority.

Acute Medical Care and Other Health Services

Critics will point out that, while the foregoing argument may provide a legitimate basis for assigning medical needs a high priority in the competition for limited social resources, it does not follow that resources assigned to health care should be spent on innovative, but very expensive, lifesaving treatments. Specifically, there may be more effective and efficient ways to reduce the impact of disease on the opportunity of persons than heavy investment in rescue interventions, such as liver transplant surgery. For example, in evaluating ways to improve the opportunity of children for a good life, we must assess the comparative impact of a liver transplant program and programs providing prenatal care, nutritional supplies, and other preventive services for children in low-income families. Proponents maintain that preventive services are much more effective and efficient in enhancing the overall health status of children than programs providing acute medical interventions.

The key issue here, however, is whether the assignment of funding priority to preventive health care services satisfies requirements of distributive justice. From this standpoint, assignment of funding priority to preventive services may be less compelling. First, the argument assumes that health care funding priorities should be assigned to services which are most effective and efficient in improving the overall health status of children. Effectiveness is construed as average improvement in health status for all children, and efficiency is interpreted as cost per unit of improvement on the effectiveness scale. But note what happens if we take this line of reasoning to its logical conclusion. It suggests that we should abandon funding support for children presently suffering from life-threatening illness for all diseases where preventive services yield a better overall payoff for health status. But most persons would be unwilling to accept this extreme implication of the argument (*cf.* Green, 1981: 158).

Second, the reason that this line of reasoning goes astray is that it fails to consider the important moral distinction already encountered between maximization and equalization of opportunity. When equalization is taken as the goal of distribution, a different assessment of the comparative worth of rescue and preventive interventions is obtained. Consider again the child who needs a liver transplant. In the absence of a transplant, the child will soon die and will be denied any opportunity for implementing his or her life plans. If societal funds available for health care are channelled into preventive programs, then the child's opportunity for a good life is completely sacrificed. By contrast, if some monies are withheld from preventive services to fund a liver transplant program, then children denied benefits of the preventive services suffer only a decline in projected health status. Equalization of opportunity requires that funding priorities be assigned to children whose medical conditions render them least well-off among potential recipients of benefits. Since the risk of death threatens opportunity more severely than the risk of decreased health status, the goal of equalizing opportunity can be best met by assigning funding priority to services for treating life-threatening health problems, such as end-state hepatic disease.

This argument in favour of assigning funding priority to services providing acute medical interventions does not require that all available funds be channelled into these services. Some preventive health programs may be more effective than acute intervention in reducing health risks for children who are medically least well-off, i.e., children whose lives are threatened by disease. For example, suppose that $500,000 is available for dealing with diseases associated with premature birth. Suppose further that it costs $25,000 per life saved to fund a neonatal intensive care unit, while it costs only $10,000 per life saved to fund free prenatal services for pregnant, low-income adolescents. If the prenatal care program can save a greater number of lives, it would receive funding priority according to the equal opportunity principle.

Nevertheless, use of the equal opportunity principle in allocation decisions will likely result in a relatively high percentage of funds for paediatric health care being devoted to acute medical interventions for life-threatening conditions. There are two reasons. One is that attention to life-threatening medical needs is more important on the equal opportunity principle than fulfillment of needs for less significant health care benefits. Since persons whose lives are at risk face greater impairment of their opportunity for a good life than persons with less serious medical needs, equalization of opportunity requires assigning priority to life-threatening needs. The other consideration is that there are many life-threatening conditions affecting children for which effective preventive strategies are not available. The basic reason is that many life-threatening childhood diseases have a much stronger genetic component and a much weaker environmental/lifestyle component than adult diseases. For example, consider the types of cancer to which children and adults are susceptible. The major childhood cancers – brain tumours, leukaemia, Wilms' tumour, neuroblastoma, osteosarcoma, etc. – originate in anatomical sites not directly affected by the environment. By contrast, major adult tumours such as lung, cervical and colon cancers occur in anatomical sites exposed to the environment. While preventive health strategies related to diet and living habits are accepted as important means for reducing the incidence of adult cancers, no similar role for prevention is workable with childhood cancer. Thus, preventive health care strategies have a less significant role than acute medical interventions in reducing the risk of death and loss of opportunities for children.

Is There a Moral Right to Innovative Therapy?

The preceding analysis suggests that three major arguments used to undercut the claim that children have a moral right to receive innovative, but very expensive lifesaving therapy are not compelling. Nevertheless, it is premature to conclude that all children with life-threatening illness have a right to receive treatment at the expense of society. There are three reasons. First, there is a limit to the claim that respect for the liberties of persons should not necessarily override the use of redistributive schemes intended to meet the basic welfare needs of other persons. The liberties denied and needs fulfilled must be weighed on a scale of moral importance. Redistribution of wealth reaches a moral limit when it conflicts with basic liberties.

Second, other basic needs and preventive programs may sometimes be more effective. Funding priority has been claimed for acute interventions over both non-medical welfare goods and preventive health care because children with life-threatening diseases are the most severely impaired with respect to their opportunity for a good life and acute interventions best increase their opportunity. Nevertheless, meeting other basic needs and implementing preventive health care programs may sometimes be more effective in rescuing children from life-threatening impairments of opportunity. Thus, funding for acute medical interventions must be carefully weighed against these other goods in determining their relative contribution to equalization of opportunity.

Third, the impact of these moral constraints on a right of children to receive innovative, but very expensive, lifesaving treatment at the expense of society must be assessed against the background of limited social resources.

Limits on resources for acute medical interventions are the product of two factors: (a) the general level of affluence in a given society; and (b) the number of children who are candidates for innovative, lifesaving treatments (Brody, 1981: 158). With medical expenditures in the United States pushing past ten percent of the gross national product, many commentators suggest that we have reached the limit of our ability to fund medical care from societal funds. This argument is rather unimpressive because the level of affluence in Western democracies appears quite extraordinary. If this point is doubted, count the number of automobiles retailing at more than thirty thousand dollars that you see in the average city during the course of one day. It takes only the cost of three of these vehicles to fund one liver transplant. If the argument is extended to include expensive, innovative care for adults as well as children, cost constraints will be more limiting. This concern is tempered by the earlier discussion of the difference between children's and adults' opportunities.

The other side of the limited resources equation is more troubling. It is not that more children are becoming candidates for lifesaving treatments as a result of a decline in general health status. Rather, more children who would have previously died are becoming candidates for acute interventions as a result of the incredible explosion of medical technology (Aaron and Schwartz, 1984). If the limits of social resources for paediatric health care are being stretched, it is more a result of the technology explosion than a result of strains upon the affluence of society.

Without attempting to estimate current limitations on societal resources due to these two factors, the following observations can be made. Insofar as these factors produce limitations, legitimate claims for liberties, non-medical goods, and preventive health care programs are placed in stiffer competition with acute medical interventions for limited resources. By legitimate claims, I mean those based upon the equal opportunity principle. Thus, the extent of the moral right of children to innovative, lifesaving treatments must be determined against the backdrop of these competing moral interests and existing limitations on resources.

Questions of effectiveness surely have to be raised when we all view the spectre of children receiving three or four livers, only ultimately to die as everyone knew would probably occur. So the problem of children's rights to innovative care is compounded by ultimate effectiveness of rapidly increasing lifesaving technologies. Unfortunately, a fledgling attempt by the Federal government in the United States to develop a serious health technology assessment program is not getting adequate support.

In the last analysis, then, this discussion has not established the conclusion that all children have a moral right to receive innovative, lifesaving treatments at the expense of society. However, the analysis has suggested that recent arguments used to discount the possibility of such a moral right are not decisive. If we take seriously the intrinsic worth of each child and the application of this commitment to distribution decisions using the principle of equal opportunity, then the medically worse-off children – those at risk from life-threatening disease – have a strong moral claim upon the resources of society. If this claim is ultimately overridden in some allocation decisions, the justification must reside in equally weighty moral considerations grounded in the equal opportunity principle. In any case, distribution of liberties, non-medical welfare goods, and preventive health care programs should not routinely preempt the provision of innovative, lifesaving therapy to children at the expense of society.

REFERENCES

Aaron, Henry and William Schwartz. 1984. *The Painful Prescription: Rationing Hospital Care*. Washington, D. C.: The Brookings Institute.

Bartholome, William. 1987. Critical commentary. Ethical issues in pediatrics conference. Calgary, Alberta.

Brody, Brauch. 1981. Health care for the haves and have nots: Toward a just basis for distribution. *Justice and Health Care*, edited by Earl Shelp. Boston: Reidel: 151-159.

Daniels, Norman. 1981. Health-care needs and distributive justice. *Philosophy and Public Affairs* 10 (Spring).

Daniels, Norman. 1985. *Just Health Care*. New York: Cambridge University Press.

Dworkin, Ronald. 1981. What is equality? Part 2: Equality of resources. *Philosophy and Public Affairs* 10 (Fall): 283-345.

Engelhardt, Jr., Tristram. 1986. *The Foundations of Bioethics*. New York: Oxford University Press.

Frankena, William. 1973. *Ethics*, 2nd Edition. Englewood Cliffs, N. J.: Prentice Hall.

Green, Ronald. 1981. Justice and the claims of future generations. *Justice and Health Care*, edited by Earl Shelp. Boston: Reidel: 194-195.

McCullough, Laurence,. 1979. The right to health care. *Ethics in Science and Medicine* 6: 1-9.

Ost, David. 1987. Critical commentary. Ethical issues in pediatrics conference. Calgary, Alberta.

Outka, Gene. 1976. Social justice and equal access to health care. *Ethics and Health Policy*, edited by Robert Veatch and Roy Branson. Cambridge, Mass.: Ballinger: 79-98.

Rawls, John. 1971. *A Theory of Justice*. Cambridge, Mass.: Harvard University Press.

Sherwin, Susan. 1984-1985. A feminist approach to ethics. *Dalhousie Review* 64 (4): 704-713.

U. S. President's Commission for the Study of Ethical Problems in Medicine and Biomedical and Behavioural Research. 1983. *Securing Access to Health Care*. Washington, D. C.: U. S. Government Printing Office.

Veatch, Robert. 1976. What is just health care delivery? *Ethics and Health Policy*, edited by Robert Veatch and Roy Branson. Cambridge, Mass.: Ballinger: 127-153.

Veatch, Robert. 1986. *The Foundations of Justice*. New York: Oxford University Press.

Mature Minors: Ethical Treatment Of Children In Medicine

Michael M. Burgess

Introduction

It is traditional to define an ethical issue by specifying the ethical principles which are in conflict. In the issue of mature minors, the conflict is between principles of beneficence, or doing good to others, and respect for persons. This is complicated in the case of children or minors, since we are uncertain of how best to respect them, and when doing good to them might conflict with such respect. I will use the term "person" to refer to the more-or-less rational, self-directing ideal of moral responsibility, partly for convenience, and because I think that there is an important notion to be protected by such a convention. I presume that any of us reading this meets the paradigm concept of what it is to be a person as an individual who can be praised and blamed for his or her actions because they are chosen from among options.

Children, at any stage of development, share in this central moral concept in two ways. First, they manifest or "possess" some of the qualities of a person. We might call this a child's current status as a person. Secondly, children have a future as autonomous beings which are more self-directing, rational and have more experience than is represented by their current state. We can call this the child's status as a developing person. So now the ethical conflict may be expressed as between seeking the child's good and respecting the child as much as the child is currently a person over and against the child as a developing person. Three general questions concretely express this ethical conflict.

58

1.   When should health care professionals and parents r[e] children's refusals? For example, it might be reasonable to accept a y[oung] child's refusal of high-risk, experimental treatment for a catastrophic dis[ease] since the chance of benefit is small and the risks are high. In such rou[tine] cases as the symptomatic treatment of a cold there may be insufficient ba[sis] to justify overruling a child's refusal of treatment.

2.   When should health care professionals accept a child's consen[t] independent of parental consent? Consider, for example, the case of [a] fourteen-year-old young woman independently requesting contraception, or a young man requesting high-risk orthopaedic surgery to improve ambulation.

3.   When should we inform children of the details of their medical condition and treatment? Specifically, when do we tell children that the experimental treatment is a last-ditch effort, that their health problem is terminal or chronic, or that the drug has certain unpleasant side effects?

The Law in Canada: Ages of Consent and the Common Law

In Canada, the age of consent is not the same as the age of majority. Rather, the age of consent to medical or surgical treatment is set by independent legislation in some provinces, and is dealt with on the basis of common law in those provinces without such legislation. In Quebec, the age of consent is fourteen, in New Brunswick and Ontario it is sixteen, and in Saskatchewan and Prince Edward Island it is eighteen. British Columbia has a legislated age of sixteen with stipulations which reduce the effectiveness of the legislation by requiring that a reasonable effort be made to contact the parents or that a written, second medical opinion be provided that the treatment is in the child's best interests (*Canadian Health Facilities Law Guide*, 1984).

The common law in Canada holds that anyone who comprehends the relevant information may consent. Lord Nathan expressed the common law position as follows:

> It is suggested that the most satisfactory solution of the problem is to rule that an infant who is capable of appreciating fully the consequences of a particular operation or of a particular treatment can give an effective consent thereto, and in such cases the consent of the guardian is unnecessary; but where the infant is without that capacity, any apparent consent

by him or her will be a nullity, the sole right to consent being vested in the guardian. (Nathan, 1957: 176)

Lorne and Faye Rozovsky, respected commentators on Canadian hospital law, suggest that legislation of ages of consent is simplistic and may be challenged on the basis of the common law (Rozovsky and Rozovsky, 1985). They recommend that medical practice should never accede to parents in order to avoid a controversy, but that the reasons underlying each party's position should be understood. Whenever it is believed that a minor is capable of deciding against a proposed procedure, even if parents are consenting, the decision of the child should be respected. They indicate that the *Canadian Charter of Rights and Freedoms* (1983) has not yet had its full impact on this area, and that any arbitrary age of consent might be struck down as discriminatory under section fifteen. They suggest that the best response is to recognize in legislation the right of a "mature minor" to give consent to all forms of health care.

I agree with the Rozovskys' recommendation, but perhaps for different reasons. I think that the legislative approach cannot specify what constitutes a mature minor for *particular* decisions, and that is precisely the critical determination for adequate responses to these problems. Therefore, the most that legislation can do is to symbolically uphold the mature minor standard, and to provide a legal basis for the prosecution of blatant abuses. Responsible parents, the public and health care professionals must develop practices which are sensitive to the relevant factors in respecting the wishes and competencies of minors. In the context of consent to, or refusal of, medical attention and treatment, a good beginning is the ethical foundations of informed consent, the basis for parental consent and what must be true for a child to be capable of giving consent or refusing treatment.

Ethical Foundations of Informed Consent

Ruth Faden and Tom Beauchamp (Faden and Beauchamp, 1986: 274-287), distinguish between two senses of informed consent. For convenience, I will label these "actual" and "institutional" informed consent. Faden and Beauchamp define an actual informed consent as an *autonomous* authorization. This has two conditions. First, the persons giving the informed consent are substantially informed and uncontrolled by external influences in their agreement. Second, they must understand that by their agreement they are authorizing a procedure which cannot proceed without such authorization.

Actual informed consent is to be distinguished from institutional consent which is defined as *effective* authorization, or authorization by a person in accordance with "operative informed consent rules in a particular policy system" (Faden and Beauchamp, 1986: 293). For example, the legislating of an age of consent stipulates specific practical circumstances in which the minor's authorization is to be accepted as valid or effective. It does not necessarily mean that all consents which do meet the age requirement of the institutional sense of informed consent will also be actual informed consents, nor will all excluded minors be incapable of actual informed consent. The institutional sense of informed consent is an attempt to standardize and operationalize the criteria of actual consent for use in institutional contexts. As Faden and Beauchamp indicate, the institutional sense of informed consent is important for the functioning of health care institutions and legal standards. But the basis for their construction, criticism and reform of such rules should be that of the actual sense of informed consent, based on the substantially autonomous person (Faden and Beauchamp, 1986: 284-287).

In other words, while the institutional or legal rules which are set up to promote informed consent cannot always guarantee actual informed consent, they ought to be designed in such a manner as to do so as much as possible. When they fail to promote actual informed consent, or impede it, that is good reason for criticism and revision. In the case of mature minors, the institutional and legal rules stipulating ages actually discourage participation of mature minors, and the sharing of information with them. In a busy schedule, health care practitioners may only take the time to share information or involve those children when they feel obliged by official policy or law. For institutional informed consent rules, the model of the autonomous person and actual informed consent is the basis for reform. For mature minors, the model of the developing autonomy of the minor and the growing ability to participate in decisions is the basis for reform.

I agree in principle with what Faden and Beauchamp have suggested and want to develop it in a manner that should be helpful for the issue of mature minors. The primary ethical role of the institutional sense of informed consent is that of a gatekeeper function (Faden and Beauchamp, 1986: 287-288), whereby those who are clearly incompetent to decide are prevented from so doing and those who are clearly competent have their "right" protected. Consequently, only the blatant abuses should be subject to institutional rules. More interesting, I think, is the role that children should play in their health care within the boundaries of the institutional rules which prohibit these extravagant abuses. This sense of actual informed consent, or the role which children should play in consent, must be based on a notion of the child as a developing autonomous person, and consequently the ethical respect due the child cannot be summarized by a discussion of informed consent. Accordingly, the remainder of the text will have three stages. First, I will examine the current institutional sense of a mature minor's role in consent. Second, I will describe the role minors may play in the actual sense of participation in authorizing. Finally, I will examine some of our ethical responsibilities in recognition of the child as a developing autonomous authorizer.

Substituted Judgment

In the absence of the ability to understand and authorize treatment of oneself, we generally substitute the consent of another person who is autonomous and will act in the patient's best interests. In the case of children, the parents or guardians are the first choice to consent on behalf of children because they are seen as having the child's best interest at heart, for reasons of parental love as well as identity of interests. I will not enter into a lengthy discussion of substituted consent, since Bill Bartholome has done an excellent job of handling the subject in his paper. While it is quite unrealistic to expect parents or professionals to project themselves "into the skin" of the child to consent on his or her behalf, it is also true that the best we can do in ascertaining what a child would want is to draw on the experiences and abilities of those closest to the child. As children are more able to participate in these discussions and decisions they ought to displace any such efforts to act on their behalf. The obvious issue which arises from this claim is just how competent must a child be in order to refuse or authorize treatment?

Variable Standards of Competency

Willard Gaylin (Gaylin, 1982), among others (Faden and Beauchamp, 1986: 288-293; Wikler, 1979; Roth, Meisel and Lidz, 1977), has argued that our criteria of competency, or the patient's ability to understand consequences of treatment and options, may be more or less stringent depending on the type of case. For some types of cases the small chance of benefit, or the temporary and incremental type of benefit, make it reasonable to consider even a young child's objection to pain or inconvenience. On the other hand, some refusals carry life-threatening implications and cannot be accepted unless the minor clearly comprehends the relevant information. According to this line of reasoning, it is more reasonable to ask how competent a minor need to be to consent or refuse a particular treatment. Or, in different words, is there any reason not to respect the minor's wishes in this particular case?

I read Gaylin to suggest that there are certain acceptable reasons for rejecting a minor's consent or refusal, but that in their absence we should respect the minor's decision.

First, if honouring the refusal or consent incurs significantly higher risk than acting contrary to the minor's wishes, then we must be sure of the minor's ability to understand the relevant information and to independently authorize or withhold authorization. Examples of this would include refusal of lifesaving treatments, such as some blood transfusions, or consent to major health risks for little or no personal or social gain, such as some clinical trials.

Second, it might be justifiable to overrule a minor's consent or refusal if the risk avoided by honouring the minor's choice is outweighed by social benefit or family integrity. So if honouring the minor's refusal to participate in an experiment of little risk but significant benefit to others creates disharmony in the family since the parents have consented, and attempts at conflict resolution have failed, it may be reasonable to overrule the minor's refusal. Gaylin suggests that to do otherwise would undercut family integrity. Most commentators agree that such conflicts ought to be worked out between parents and children. I would add the stipulation that if the minor is quite mature, and the difference seems to be one of differing value choices, the investigator or practitioner would be wise to respect the minor's wishes.

Third, when very young children refuse or object to experimental or therapeutic procedures they may be overruled by parents on the basis that the parents have the authority to determine their children's education and socialization. As many authors have noted (Bartholome, 1977), justification of (low-risk) research on the basis of moral development is only valid in the case of children who are old enough to understand the moral implications of their actions.

We have identified three types of minors' participation in medical treatment and research. The most basic level is the refusal of a medical procedure, perhaps on the basis of pain, anxiety or inconvenience. The procedure must not be one which is of significant gain to the child. This refusal could be overruled by parents, although it would be best to talk to the child to alleviate anxieties and reduce distrust.

The second level of participation in consent is when minors have sufficient cognitive development to understand the relevant information, at least the basic information, and on that basis may agree to, or refuse a medical procedure. It will be rare that children at this stage will disagree with parents, and those that do should have the issues discussed so that they understand the basis for pursuing or avoiding the medical procedure. Procedures which are high risk, even if high gain, such as experimental cardiac surgery with a high mortality rate, should certainly be explained to these minors and their assent is necessary. If they refuse the treatment, their understanding should be verified, and, if they cannot be persuaded to assent, their refusal should probably be taken as binding for these procedures. Furthermore, consent to low-risk, high-gain procedures such as blood transfusions may be taken as sufficient, but refusals should be carefully examined for competence and independence of thought. A high risk of loss of life is a good basis to challenge a minor's refusal or consent at this level.

The third level is when the minor is mature enough to comprehend the relevant information and independent enough to realize what is implied by an act of authorizing. Consents and refusals are all ethically binding in these cases, except under the same mitigating circumstances to which competent adults are subject.

Thus far I have avoided mention of ages, in part out of concern that the tendency to use ages as definitive of maturity is too convenient and overshadows the more important discussion of development and maturity. But without age groupings, this discussion is without concrete markers to guide the application of recommendations. I am not convinced that any age should be part of institutional policy or legislation, and even there I have reservations. Age categories should merely serve as rules of thumb to guide practice by alerting us to be sensitive to developing competencies and abilities.

Numerous studies which are referred to in Sanford Leiken's excellent paper for the President's Commission (Leiken, 1982) have shown that cognitive development and performance is affected by a variety of factors independent of age (cf. Melton, Koocher, and Saks, 1983; Grisso and Vierling, 1978; Melton, 1980). Children of the same age but different social classes show different levels of development (Melton, 1980). Social setting influences not only the child's rate of development, but also each performance, so that a minor may appear much more mature in a home than in a hospital, or when in the presence of parents than without. Some children are more independent when away from their parents and the physician (Grisso and Vierling, 1978; Melton, 1980). Healthy children seem to perform better than do sick children of the same age, but chronically ill children sometimes outperform both (Cook, 1975; Brewster, 1982). I mention this only to emphasize that age groupings are very poor predictors of performance and that the application of such generalizations should be quite tentative so as not to be prejudicial. Age categories should not be used simply out of convenience or to avoid conflict.

Sanford Leiken (Leiken, 1982) utilizes Piaget's model of cognitive development (Piaget, 1952) to examine children's competency for consent (cf. Bibace and Walsh, 1980; Warner, 1948). He suggests that around seven to ten years there is a major shift in the child's emphasis of the difference between self and others. Prior to this stage of development, the child conceives illness as caused by proximity or magic and healing as a matter of obeying rules. So at this earlier stage of development, the child's refusals are likely based on dislike or misconceptions, rather than any understanding of the illness or medical procedures. But the seven- to ten-year-old child perceives illness as caused by contamination, and there is greater differentiation of self from others, so the child is now more likely to understand some of the basic information about the illness and treatment and so be able to have some rational, although possibly misconceived, basis for refusing or agreeing to the procedure (Leiken, 1982: 181-182). Refusals should certainly be overruled only with careful explanations, and agreement to treatment should be sought, although the child should not be thought to be capable of authorizing treatment.

Around eleven years, with the development of formal-logical thinking, there is the greatest differentiation of self and others. The child's concept of illness is one of multiple causes, with a sense of the body's defensive responses (Leiken, 1982: 180-181). From this time on, the minor's choice should only be overruled with careful explanation, and such rejection must be justified on ethical grounds, such as those mentioned above. From eleven to fourteen years of age is a very transitional state, and these minors should be treated under the second or third level, where the minor's agreement is required for treatment, and their consent is sufficient for low-risk, high-gain medical procedures. Practically speaking, it will be rare for a child of this age to desire to consent to treatment independent of parents, but when they are independent enough to do so that should be taken as reason to evaluate whether they have developed to the point of a mature minor with full "rights of consent."

At about fourteen years of age the minor is likely to have developed sufficient cognitive capacity to understand carefully explained medical information and enough independence and self-awareness to authorize in his or her own behalf. This means that their consents should be taken as sufficient, their refusals binding and their parents' proxy consents as either irrelevant or at least insufficient without the minor's informed consent. These are, of course, subject to the same limitations of the informed consent of competent adults, such as absence of undue influence.

Autonomy as a Developmental Goal

Note that throughout the stages of development my emphasis has been on respecting whatever cognitive development and independent thinking the child has developed. Respect for the child's developing capacities and involvement in medical decisions also should encourage the maturation of the child. Since the focus of this paper is respecting the existing and the developing person in the child, the final portion will deal with how, in medical practice, we can further respect the child's developing autonomy.

Whether we are dealing with children or adults, informed consent is never an ethically sufficient doctrine. No set of institutional rules can guarantee actual valid consent in every case, and even in cases of actual consent there are other ethical issues which may arise (e.g., otherwise it would not make sense to speak of the possibility of valid consent to immoral actions). The emphasis on informed consent in medical ethics has increased an already strong tendency to deal with ethics in a legalistic, contractual manner which requires the establishment of claims to moral rights. Feminist ethics have helped us to understand that we would do better to consider the responsibilities of persons in the context of relationships rather than focusing on the establishment of the rights of isolated persons (*cf.* Sherwin, 1985; Noddings, 1984). Furthermore, informed consent has only dealt with the conflict between the moral values of doing good to others and their self-direction. But as children mature, we do recognize that they have responsibilities and that other values become relevant in judging their actions. That is why we hold juvenile offenders responsible for their actions and praise the "good citizenship" of even elementary school children.

The justification of low-risk, non-therapeutic research on children based on their gain in terms of moral development is now fairly widely accepted (McCormick, 1974; Pence, 1980; Gaylin, 1982: 37). This is based on the idea that it is justifiable to expose children to risks for gain to others as long as the children benefit in some significant manner. So we tend to accept as ethical some research on children which was once thought to be clearly unethical. The justification of children's participation in this research is based on four presuppositions which must be reasonable in each case.

First, we assume that such moral development is important. Second, we must have good reason to believe that the child has the capacity to benefit in this manner. Third, the child's participation is likely to result in such moral development. Fourth, there must not be a significant increase of risk over that of everyday activities and recreation. Inasmuch as the developing child is capable of such social contributions, it is not unreasonable to offer parents and children this opportunity for the nurturance of positive social attitudes.

Respect and nurturance of the developing person suggests that it is appropriate to consider information disclosure, social and emotional support, individualized explanation and whatever involvement the child is capable of. Even very young children may benefit emotionally and psychologically from efforts to communicate and support their expressions of anxiety, fear, trust and hope. Furthermore, as the child matures, initial support and communication may provide an opportunity for the assessment and enhancement of the child's ability to participate in decisions. There are also ways to increase children's ability to participate or perform at a higher level, thereby respecting their current capacities and encouraging their development. Parental and peer involvement seems to increase children's ability to understand and think (Grisso and Vierling, 1978; Melton, 1980). Continuity of care is important as well, inasmuch as the child is highly responsive to trust which can build over time in a supportive relationship.

Conclusion

Out of respect of the developing person, and the person as developed thus far, we should always attempt to inform children of their condition and treatments. The emphasis should be on emotional support and on building a trusting relationship. This may also increase the child's ability to express desires or choices, thus to begin to participate in their health care. In this manner, an opportunity is also provided for the assessment of comprehension and ability to authorize, which can serve as a safeguard against inappropriate dependence on age limits. A child's refusal or opposition should always be respected in that it should not be casually overruled merely because it is a child's action. The first effort ought to be an attempt to understand the basis for the child's opposition. Serious efforts should be made to respect the child's basis for refusal, whether through discussion or accepting the refusal. Practitioners and parents should talk to the child to better understand the opposition and to gain the child's trust. Overruling the opposition of a child is a violation of such trust and must be carefully justified on the basis of low risk and high benefit, low risk and child's best interests, or high social good (e.g., contagious disease control). The basis for overruling the child's refusal should be explained to the child, or at least the child should be emotionally supported by parents and practitioners at each action or procedure which reinforces the fact of being overruled. A child's consent is independently sufficient if the child is capable of understanding the nature of the procedure and its consequences, as well as that of the options. Consent of children just below this level of ability should be considered sufficient only if the procedure is low risk and of considerable personal or social benefit. In this manner we can respect the developing person, encourage the development of ethical values, promote autonomy and social welfare as values, and allow children their proper role as consenting patients and subjects.

So in general everyday delivery of health care, the child ought to be given a more active role, starting with strong emotional support and attention to expressions of opposition and moving to a greater attempt to communicate to the child his or her health status and the implications of treatments selected on the child's behalf. This involvement should escalate as the child manifests the ability to understand the information. High-risk and low-gain procedures, or low-risk, low-gain procedures must have the assent of any capable child. Finally, we should endeavour to reduce the frequency and institutional sanction of the rejection of mature minor consents which are given by comprehending and independent persons who happen to fall below an arbitrary legal age.

REFERENCES

Bartholome, W. 1977. Parents, children and the moral benefits of research. *National Commission for the Protection of Human Subjects of Biomedical and Behavioral Research. Appendix: Research Involving Children.* DHEW Publication No. OS 77-00055. Reprinted in T. A. Mappes and J. S. Zemabaty (editors), *Biomedical Ethics* (First Edition). New York: McGraw-Hill, 1981: 169-172.

Bibace, R. and M. Walsh. 1980. Development of children's concept of illness. *Pediatrics* 66: 912-917.

Brewster, A. 1982. Chronically ill hospitalized children's concepts of their illness. *Pediatrics* 19: 355-362.

Canadian Health Facilities Law Guide. 1984. Don Mills, Ontario: Commerce Clearing House, Inc.: 1147-1161.

Canadian Charter of Rights and Freedoms. 1983. Canadian Institute for the Administration of Justice. Quebec: Editions Yvon Blais.

Cook, S. 1975. The development of causal thinking with regard to physical illness among French children. Thesis, University of Kansas, Kansas City. (As reported in S. Leiken, 1982.)

Faden, R. R. and T. L. Beauchamp. 1986. *A History and Theory of Informed Consent.* New York: Oxford University Press.

Gaylin, W. 1982. The competence of children: No longer all or none. *The Hastings Center Report* 12, No. 2: 33-38.

Gaylin, W. and R. Macklin. 1982. *Who Speaks for the Child.* New York: Plenum Press.

Grisso, T. and L. Vierling. 1978. Minors' consent to treatment: A developmental perspective. *Professional Psychology* (August, 1978): 412-426.

Leiken, S. L. 1982. Minors' assent or dissent. *Making Health Care Decisions. Volume Three: Appendices: Studies on the Foundations of Informed Consent.* President's Commission for the Study of Ethical Problems in Medicine and Biomedical and Behavioral Research. Washington, D. C.: U. S. Government Printing Office: 174-191.

McCormick, R. A. 1974. Proxy consent in the experimentation situation. *Perspectives in Biology and Medicine* 18, No. l: 2-20.

Melton, G. B. 1980. Children's concepts of their rights. *Journal of Clinical Psychology* 9: 186-190.

Melton, G. B., G. P. Koocher, and M. J. Saks (editors). 1983. *Children's Competence to Consent.* New York: Plenum Press.

Nathan, Lord. 1957. *Medical Negligence.* London: Butterworth's. As reprinted in *The Canadian Health Facilities Law Guide*, 1984: 1148.

70

Noddings, Nel. 1984. *Caring*. Berkeley: University of California Press.

Pence, G. E. 1980. Children's dissent to research – a minor matter? *IRB: A Review of Human Subjects Research* 2 (December 1980): 1-4.

Piaget, J. 1952. *The Origins of Intelligence in Children*. New York: International University's Press.

Roth, L., A. Meisel, and C. W. Lidz. 1977. Tests of competency to consent to treatment. *American Journal of Psychiatry* 134: 279-285.

Rozovsky, L. E. and F. A. Rozovsky. 1985. Do you know the *real* age of consent? *Canadian Doctor*, February, 1985: 53-55.

Sherwin, S. 1984-1985. A feminist approach to ethics. *Dalhousie Review* 64 (4): 704-713.

Warner, H. 1948. *Comparative Psychology of Mental Development*. New York: Science Editions.

Wikler, D. 1979. Paternalism and the mildly retarded. *Philosophy and Public Affairs* 8: 377-392.

Non-Treatment and Non-Compliance as Neglect

Susan Sherwin

Neglect: to give little or no attention or respect to: consider or deal with as if of little or no importance: to fail to attend to sufficiently or properly: not give proper attention or care to: to carelessly omit doing (something that should be done)...leave unattended to through carelessness: pass lightly over.

– Webster's Third International Dictionary (Unabridged)

Western society has made considerable progress over the centuries in our protection of the interests of children. We no longer have laws declaring children to be the private property of their father who can kill, sell, or use them however he chooses, as Roman law decreed under *patria potestas*. Current laws explicitly restrict the authority of parents over their children and make parents liable to abuse and neglect. Both the Criminal Code of Canada and provincial child welfare acts govern the obligation of parents to ensure that their children receive the necessities of life. Laws authorizing state intervention if parents are found to be inadequate guardians are relatively recent, though, and their interpretation and scope remain unclear. But they clearly reflect a marked change in social attitude: children are increasingly viewed as vulnerable persons with rights and interests to be protected, rather than as private property to be used as the parents decide (Dickens, 1984).

We still have a long way to go, however, if we are truly interested in protecting the welfare of children. Far too many Canadian children die each year from severe abuse and neglect. Emergency room doctors see thousands of children who have been brutalized and tortured by their parents or caretakers. Moreover, there is evidence that millions of Canadian children are victims of sexual abuse: in his important study, Robin Badley concluded that more than half the girls and one third of the boys in this country are sexually abused as children (Badley, 1984). Even within the family, supposedly the seat of greatest concern for the child, evidence suggests that at least sixteen percent of Canadian girls experience incestuous abuse before the age of eighteen, including four and a half percent by their fathers (Russell, 1986). Though such treatment of children is prohibited by law, only a tiny proportion of cases are identified, and only a few of these are prosecuted. For most purposes, parents are still allowed enormous control over their children.

These disturbing statistics reflect an area of concern for anyone who cares about the welfare of children. For those involved in paediatrics, there is particular anguish, since people who work in this area are usually personally committed to the well-being of children. Further, their work makes it especially likely that they shall be the ones to discover evidence of the mistreatment of children. For this reason, they are legally charged with the responsibility to report suspected abuse to authorities who might attempt to redress the situation. I consider it quite proper that those involved in delivering health care to children be on the lookout for cases of physical, sexual, or psychological abuse, and for cases of gross neglect of the necessities of life, including adequate food, clothing, shelter and health care.

When abuse or serious neglect is identified, it is important for the authorities concerned to make an effort to identify the source of the problem, since many diverse explanations are possible, and each requires a different response. The mistreatment may be a result of genuine neglect as defined by *Webster's* above, i.e., it may reflect a failure to value the child appropriately, and, hence, inadequate attention is paid to her/his welfare. But it may also reflect ignorance of the child's real needs: for example, child sexual abuse can sometimes be explained by the perpetrator's ignorance of the harm such activity causes the child.[1] In contrast, the absence of

---

[1] This is not altogether surprising in light of the many reported statements by sexuality experts which rationalize such treatment by suggesting that adult-child sexual experiences are actually beneficial to the child. The Kinsey study, for instance, dismissed the proposition that sexual

necessities is often a result of the parent's inability to obtain adequate resources. Housing, for instance, is a chronic problem for low-income families, and government support through social services is frequently too low to ensure proper care for children. Parents in such circumstances feel helpless: they do not like to complain about inadequate support, since they fear losing custody of their children if they admit that they cannot provide properly for their needs. The legal terms of "abuse" and "neglect" are not appropriate for addressing this entire range of cases.

In medical contexts, the concepts of abuse and neglect should be used only in a restricted set of cases. Abuse might be involved in the event of disturbing and unnecessary medical intervention, such as painful testing in a case where there is virtually no hope, and some authors would consider instances of medical experimentation with children as constituting abuse. In most cases which I consider to be instances of medical abuse, the physician plays an important role either by initiating the questionable treatment or by complying with parental demands that more be done despite the physician's clear judgment that further treatment will be far more likely to harm than to help the child. There are surely a few cases where the parent(s) can be seen as the primary source of medical abuse, e.g., in the case of Kevin Starke, documented by Berton Roueche (1986), who was a victim of what has been termed the "Munchausen Syndrome by Proxy": his mother brought him to a paediatrician for frequent (weekly) medical treatment, reporting non-existent symptoms which were then treated with tests and drugs. To be sure, some parents are overly anxious and will seek unnecessary medical care, but the incidence of parents deliberately fabricating illnesses for their children in an effort to obtain unneeded treatment appears to be extremely rare. Only these latter exceptional cases should be considered as abuse.

Cases of suspected neglect seem far more common. Again these include cases of neglect on the part of medical practitioners where appropriate treatment is not provided, usually because of incompetence,

---

contacts with children are damaging to the child, and in *Penthouse* in 1976, Wardell Pomeroy, one of the authors of the Kinsey study wrote, "Incest between adults and younger children can also prove to be a satisfying and enriching experience although difficulties can certainly arise." (Russell, 1986: 8).

negligence, or poor communication. Occasionally, other factors can interfere with provision of proper medical service, e.g., financial restraints or organized protests (such as in a strike situation or work-to-rule campaign). Health professional organizations prefer to deal with at least the former sorts of cases through internal discipline committees, viewing them as isolated anomalies. Some people would add cases of selective non-treatment, where the medical staff judge that a child's prognosis is so poor that medical treatment is inappropriate, as another area of neglect.

From the medical point of view, however, the most common instances of neglect on medical matters are described as failures in responsibility on the part of the parents. In other words, the invocation of the blame-laden term "neglect" is generally reserved for parents. It is important to note that both non-treatment and non-compliance, the two types of failure to which I have been invited to address, are defined from the medical perspective: that is, doctors choose the preferred treatment regimen, and, if parents fail to comply, their behavior is labelled as constituting non-treatment or non-compliance. These are terms which function as criticism of parental failure to accept and follow authoritative advice. They can only be applied to medical staff if some other medical authority defines treatment norms which they defy.

The most notorious cases where non-treatment is a concern are those involving neonates with severe birth defects, a subject mentioned in earlier papers. In those cases, the paediatricians involved usually make a preliminary judgment as to what sort of treatment is available and whether or not there is any reasonable likelihood that the infant may benefit from that treatment. If they determine that there is no promising therapy and the condition is hopeless, they will generally report that tragic news to the parents and support them through the period of dying, offering only palliative care to the baby. If, however, they identify a treatment that may extend the life of the infant, and especially if they recognize one that has some hope of improving the prospects for that infant, they will generally report that information to the parent(s) and request permission to commence treatment. Only in these cases, where medical treatment is recommended by the specialists, would a parental decision to reject that therapy be labelled as constituting neglect. If the doctors and parents concur that the prospects for therapy are so dismal as to make a negative decision seem justified, then judgmental terms are not invoked. But if, in contrast, medical opinion supports initiating treatment, then medical staff are likely to feel anger and frustration with recalcitrant parents, seeing them to be failing in their obligation to provide for the well-being of their children. In such cases, it has proved to be extremely tempting to seek legal recourse by securing limited guardianship in order to ensure treatment.

Coercive, legal solutions seem to be insensitive to the fact that decisions about treatment for severely defective newborns are terribly difficult. Caring, ethical persons with the best will in the world are capable of disagreeing about what is best for some of these children. There are a variety of values in conflict in these situations, including the value of preserving life, the expected quality of life, individual attitudes toward risk-taking, the burden of caring for the child, and the effects of that care on others. The anguish is particularly acute when, as in a significant number of cases, there is no certainty about the long-term consequences for the child and a significant likelihood of making things worse through treatment.

Under such circumstances, it is not surprising that there will be cases where the individuals involved with a child's care will have serious differences about the appropriate treatment in some particular case. One may favour aggressive treatment and another may prefer only palliative care, yet both may be working from the same moral principle of beneficence. Hence, while agreeing that the child's interest is paramount, adults may come to radically different conclusions about the suitability of therapy. Physicians, health care workers, hospitals, bioethicists, judges, and politicians have wrestled with such issues for many years now, and no universally acceptable criteria are apparent. For many types of cases, no consensus exists as to what action is the right one. When parents and doctors disagree about the care of a newborn, it is highly probable that the party who seeks treatment will judge the reluctant party to be neglecting the welfare of that child. Such a judgment is simply false in many of these hard cases: the other party may be equally or even more concerned with the welfare of the child than the one who seeks to implement treatment, but makes a different evaluation of what constitutes the best interest of that child. Under such circumstances, it would be wrong and insulting to employ the apparatus of legal neglect to coerce the other into compliance. Another solution must be sought if (but only if) there are reasonable grounds for uncertainty about where the child's best interests lie.

Similar problems arise with older children facing life-threatening illnesses. It is perfectly understandable that parents occasionally deny a terminal diagnosis for their child and insist that the specialists pursue additional tests and experimental therapies despite medical advice that there is no prospect of success. Where the medical staff despair of the benefit of such therapy and recognize the importance of reducing the child's discomfort and alienation, parents may insist on further measures in a frantic attempt at a final miracle and consider the staff negligent if they refuse to proceed. Should time and finances permit, they could probably find some expert somewhere who would support their conviction that there is more to be done and that the initial doctors were irresponsible in not attempting this treatment. The child may well suffer additionally from this pursuit, increasing the degree of tragedy facing her.

Most doctors protect themselves against such charges by adopting an attitude of trying everything possible, no matter how remote the likelihood of saving the life. It has been widely acknowledged that physicians do not like to accept death and consider it a personal defeat, especially when dealing with children. Parents, too, hate to admit that their child will die, but they also hate to watch the child suffer, and they feel alienated and distant from the child in hospital. If they do not expect that the child's condition can be cured, and if they believe that continued survival constitutes a serious burden of suffering on that child, they will sometimes deny permission for continued therapy and seek to have the child "left in peace." Such sentiments on behalf of loving parents are again understandable; many health care workers have been known to echo them. In fact, physicians, surveyed on Canadian practices with sick newborns admitted that they would decide differently if acting as parents than they do when acting as physicians (Magnet and Kluge, 1985: 25). Nonetheless, those who wish to pursue every option refuse to ignore any chance of survival, however remote, and they may well judge parents negligent if they do not provide their child with this last chance. Again, I would consider the determination of neglect, and, in particular, the legal apparatus of charges of neglect to be the wrong means for addressing this sort of disagreement.

In cases where the odds are slightly better, the uncertainty may be even more acute. What if the child's survival chances are not unprecedented, but more likely twenty percent, and his ultimate condition would not be overwhelmingly burdensome? I doubt if any doctors would deny therapy under such circumstances, but some parents still would, particularly if they judged the discomfort of the therapy to be extreme. Since many adult patients make these sorts of decisions for themselves, it is not necessarily wrong to make such a choice paternalistically on behalf of another. If four out of five children die after a painful and terrifying number of months of chemotherapy, it would not be evidence of neglect if parents choose not to hospitalize the child for what is likely to be its remaining months, but instead head off with the rest of the family for a week in Disney World. It is an agonizing choice for loving, concerned parents, and for caring physicians: yet, if, in weighing up the values, we opt for a chance at more life even at the expense of hazardous and distressing therapy, I think it would be improper to use blame-loaded terms like "neglect" to express our frustration. (Conversely, we should refrain from labelling those who favour treatment as being guilty of abuse.)

But there are cases, and there are cases. Sometimes the child has a very good, even a virtually certain chance of recovery, yet the parents may still refuse therapy. Under these sorts of circumstances, we would need to know more about the reasons for refusal before we could consider it a case of neglect. I would agree that it is an instance of neglect if the parents simply do not want the child and wish it dead, e.g., if it was born with a handicap, such as Down's syndrome, which they cannot accept, or if it was the wrong sex (infanticide of girls is still practiced in various locations on the globe), or if it cried too much and was a general nuisance. I would also consider it neglect if the parents simply could not be bothered to see to it that proper care was received, or if they were unwilling to reschedule a vacation so that therapy could begin.[2] If, however, the therapy is refused for religious reasons, either because the parents' religion refuses all medical intervention, or just the particular therapy at hand, I think it is again inappropriate to try to categorize such cases under the rubric of neglect. In these last cases, the refusal is not based on neglect for the child's welfare, but on a disagreement of values about what constitutes that welfare.

Jehovah's Witnesses' parents who refuse blood transfusions are not indifferent to the child's well-being: they just appeal to different evidence to define it. Current practice dictates that the courts ensure transfer of limited guardianship to allow the prescribed blood therapy, but I suggest that this approach be used cautiously. As Terrence Ackerman argued in "The Limits of Beneficence," there are circumstances where it is wrong to insist on transfusions over parental objection, even if the child might benefit (Ackerman, 1980). With certain cancers, recovery prospects may be poor, treatment regimens are often long and may produce harmful side-effects, and dealing with a life-threatening illness tends to create great stress for the patient and family; hence, it is extremely important to develop and protect trusting relationships among the patient, parents and medical team. Obviously, court-ordered transfusions may compromise such a relationship, and Ackerman (1980: 18) recommends that we not seek them automatically, but that we override the parental decision "only if the intervention is more likely than not to prevent the degree of substantial harm that will be caused by the parental action itself." If we acknowledge that when "the probability of indefinite, disease-free survival is less than 50 percent, further cancer therapy is more likely to result in a greater degree of harm than non-treatment (Ackerman, 1980: 17), we can see that intervening in the face of parental refusal will frequently be unacceptable, especially on grounds of neglect.[3]

---

[2] A recent Toronto case appears to constitute a paradigm example of medical neglect: apparently parents of a five-year-old boy with Hischsprung's disease, a curable condition involving severe constipation, did not obtain medical assistance and the child suffered a prolonged suffering death. The police have chosen to prosecute the parents for manslaughter in this case (*The Globe and Mail*, 1987).

[3] The Ontario Provincial Court (Family Division) seems to have reached a similar conclusion (November 1, 1985) when it denied the application of the Children's Aid Society for a

But uncertainty is a chronic problem in medicine, especially in paediatric medicine. Some parents believe they love their children too much to allow expensive, technological, risky treatments to be used: others are indignant when heroic measures are not taken. We can accuse neither of neglecting their child, and I believe that the state has no moral authority to overrule either decision when no one can say with justifiable confidence which way the child will be better off.

Transfer of decision-making authority is appropriate only when there is authoritative technical information establishing that the child is more likely to be significantly benefited one way rather than the other. Even so, determinations of neglect should only be invoked here if there is also some clear independent evidence that the parents are not sufficiently interested in the child's welfare. Otherwise, if the definition of where the child's welfare lies is not clear, or if the parents demonstrate an active concern with the child's condition, I suggest that we allow the parents the freedom to decide according to their best judgment of where the child's interests reside, with advice from whomever they choose.

Similar problems occur when we turn to the area of non-compliance, except that here the labelling goes even more routinely in only one direction.[4] Compliance and its omission are defined by the medical professionals. Patients, or, in the case of children, parents, are the ones judged guilty of non-compliance whenever they do not follow through on "doctor's orders." By definition here, non-compliance is a term understood to attribute fault in the form of irresponsibility. It is well known that only a fraction of adult patients are fully compliant with their own medical regimens (Cohen, 1979), so we should not be surprised to find a high degree of non-compliant behaviour in dealing with children. Again, it is necessary to

---

declaration that a twelve-year-old Jehovah's Witness child with fatal leukemia disease was in need of protection: the parents and child objected to routine chemotherapy and blood transfusions with a thirty percent rate of cure, preferring to pursue mega-vitamin therapy (*Canadian Family Law Guide*, 1985: 4915).

[4]Non-compliance by physicians has been defined as including failure to report tests to patients, following up on symptoms reported, scheduling tests, and notifying patients of new findings on their condition or therapy (L. V. Pratt, 1982: 251). Leon Gordis defines it as failure of the physician to "comply with current expert opinion" (Gordis, 1979: 43).

consider the circumstances that lead up to such apparently negative behaviour.

Sometimes, I am sure, non-compliance is indeed a reflection of neglect. The child's parents or caretakers simply do not care enough for the welfare of the child to ensure that therapeutic regimens are followed. Far more commonly, however, are cases where something less blameworthy is operating. It may be that the parent really is incapable of providing responsible care. He may be suffering from an alcohol or drug-addiction problem, or from depression or schizophrenia: any of these conditions might interfere with his ability to provide proper attention to his children. In that case, there would be grounds for intervention to assure that the child's health needs are being met, but again I would urge caution in invoking the label of neglect, for mental illness and alcoholism do not necessarily prove that one is an uncaring or unfit parent.

Alternatively, non-compliance may occur because the parent does not have the resources to ensure treatment: she may just not be able to afford the medications or the taxi to the clinic, take the time for follow-up sessions, or spend time monitoring the child's progress at home. Often, poor communication will result in misunderstanding so that the parent does not really understand the obligation for continuing care. There will also be cases where another opinion is offered and the parent finds that proposal more agreeable, even if it is coming from an unauthorized source. None of these latter cases constitute neglect, for the parents are quite attentive to the interests of the child: they are just mistaken about how best to protect them or are lacking the means to do so. Seeking legal redress against such parents is unlikely to help much: other, more cooperative solutions must be found, such as better social support, more care taken in communication, and explicit justification of the recommended therapy.

Often, non-compliance is an indication of no real agreement in the first place. Adult patients and guardians of the non-competent have a legal and moral right to consent to treatment. For that consent to be valid, it should be informed and voluntary. Parents, like adult patients, often do not believe they are fully informed of their options, and they often feel very intimidated by the medical context and hence express insincere agreement to things without any real commitment. Sartre may consider such disingenuousness to constitute bad faith, but most of us can understand the motivation. "Consent" tends to be regarded as the right to agree with the doctor's direction, but not to choose alternatives or even really to refuse. Adult patients who refuse to consent run the risk of having their mental competence challenged: parents who wish to refuse run the risk of having their competence as guardians thrown into question.

Yet there may be good reasons for not consenting. In pondering the uncertainties and conflicting values at stake in medical decision-making, it is not apparent that the expert's willingness to take one risk should overrule a parent's wish to take another. Ideally, we leave those weighings to the patient, since she is the person likely to be most profoundly affected by the outcome; in other words, we recognize that decisions about medical care are fundamentally private matters. Hence, it is very important to ascertain the wishes of older children. Young children, obviously, cannot choose for themselves, so someone must offer their substituted judgment on their behalf. In the competition for who chooses for them, I believe the rule should be *ceteris paribus*, to give priority to the person(s) most likely to have the strongest regard for the child. Generally, that will be whomever is involved in the longest and deepest relationship with that child – usually the parents. Hence, with compliance as with treatment, barring evidence of other forms of neglect or clear indication that the medical course will be significantly more beneficial to the child, the parents' decision should be respected.

Parents have a right to have their decisions respected in these circumstances, not because they always make the best choices for their children – they don't – but because, other things being equal, they are more likely to act in accordance with their child's interests than any other individual or institution. Like democracy, parental authority is an imperfect system for decision-making, but it is the least imperfect system available.

In defending parents' rights to choose, I do not wish to endorse lingering social attitudes that children are in any sense the property of their parents. I do not believe that parents have the right to do as they like with their children. As a society, we continue to be ambivalent about the status of children and their relation to their parents. To a large extent, we still think of children as a sort of property of their parents. Parents are held to be responsible for a child's welfare and behaviour, and have a great deal of freedom on how that child shall be raised. Rather than recognizing that children constitute a social benefit and burden, there is a strong tendency to continue to privatize them like property. Children who remain "unclaimed," because they are too handicapped, too disturbed, the wrong race, or the wrong age are neglected by society. Tens of thousands of children are caught on a treadmill of shifting, unsatisfactory foster homes which, in the majority of cases, do not meet their emotional needs, and sometimes barely meet their physical needs. Many "unowned" teenagers are now slipping through the cracks where no placement can be found for them outside the juvenile justice system. And, should we consider looking outside of our own borders, we find millions of children dying for want of basic food or simple, inexpensive inoculation and health care measures. If, as a society, we really care about protecting the life and health of children, I would think it would be most appropriate to begin attending to children suffering genuine neglect, either by their parents, their community, or their state (or a combination thereof). That is the appropriate sphere for *parens patriae.*

Discussion in medical ethics focuses on compelling parents to consent to expensive, imposing, aggressive therapy for children who may not survive in a state which most people recognize as human. At the same time, as a society, we abandon all these other potentially healthy children. This disparity in concern about the welfare of distinct populations of children suggests that we must look deeper into the underlying values governing these discussions. A general, principled concern for neglected children does not seem to account for this inconsistency in the focus of our attention.

Children whose parents make a caring, if mistaken judgment about their medical treatment are not neglected, especially when considered in the context of society's own abandonment of children with more desperate, if less technical, needs. This may be hard to accept for those involved in paediatric medicine, since, after all, it is usually only the former sort of children who are brought to their attention. A child who is genuinely neglected is far less likely to find her way to specialized medical care than one who has a concerned and attentive caretaker.[5] Yet, it is just the latter sort of guardian who is likely to want to make an independent judgment about the child's best interests, and hence, may be unwilling to merely accept expert advice passively. In many cases, disagreement with medical advice is a reflection of caring and not neglect. Hence, a general concern to protect the interests of neglected children would not begin with those whose parents' active involvement in decision-making about their child's medical care results in disagreement with the particular medical authorities they encounter.

I believe that the state has a far greater responsibility than it now accepts in protecting the interests of children who are abused or neglected, and that health care personnel have an important role to play in fulfilling that responsibility. Parents who are sadistic, dangerous, or indifferent to their children have no right to mistreat their children simply because they are "theirs" in some sense. In many cases, we as a society tend to be far too unwilling to interfere with "sanctity of the family," so we stand by and allow children to be damaged beyond repair by parental mistreatment.

Refusal of medical advice, however, is not, in and of itself, evidence of neglect. It is very presumptuous to declare that medical values override a family's values, especially when medical success cannot be assured. The conflict created by the imposition of pejorative labels like "neglect," especially if legal action is then taken against the parents, is certain to weaken the bonds of trust between the child's permanent and medical caretakers. This result will be costly to the child's security and support system, and is likely to complicate compliance problems later.

We should be giving much greater weight to the significance of trust in medical relationships than has been done to date. In hard medical cases, there is a tendency to limit our focus to medical facts. The bioethics literature has encouraged us to broaden our scope to include moral considerations as well as medical ones in value decisions, but most of that literature includes a restricted list of moral criteria. The leading candidates are respect for individual autonomy (which underlies commitment to

---

[5]This is true only for children beyond the age of perinatal care. For hospital-born newborns (as most Canadian babies are), referral to neonatal units is usually taken unilaterally by attending physicians with minimal parental involvement (Magnet and Kluge, 1985: 9-16).

informed consent) and the principle of beneficence (which urges us to refrain from harming, and seek to benefit patients). Concern for justice is included when resource allocation decisions must be made, and some authors insist on a baseline commitment to respecting the sanctity of life. These values constitute the core of the dominant ethical theories which most philosophers currently endorse, but, along with a growing number of other philosophers, I object to this traditionally defined agenda; I think other values should be recognized as central to moral decision-making (Sherwin, 1984-1985: 705; Forthcoming). Nel Noddings, for instance, has argued for a view of ethics based entirely on interpersonal relationships of caring (Noddings, 1984). Annette Baier has been developing an approach to ethics based on trust (and anti-trust), which is particularly salient in this context (Baier, 1985; 1986). In Baier's view, trust is a central moral consideration which merits principal ethical attention. She argues that trust is essential in all human enterprises, but that it cannot and should not be extended uncritically. It is easily abused, and for that reason, is highly fragile.

Ideally, and frequently in practice, health professionals are trusted to use their expertise in identifying the best interests of their patients. Further, society as a whole implicitly trusts most parents to act in accordance with their child's interest. Yet in recent years, both sorts of trust have been eroding. Numerous public accounts of negligence, incompetence, and exploitation by individual physicians have undermined many people's blanket trust in their doctors. Medical horror stories abound, and many have had unsatisfactory relationships with the medical establishment. Chilling stories of child abuse have also led us to be far more cautious in our reliance on parents to protect children's interests. In such a climate, it is not hard to understand why, in many instances, a relationship between parents of dangerously ill children and health workers may have shifted from one of mutual reliance and cooperative support to an adversarial contest, even though a good trusting relationship between parents and doctors is extremely important in the care of children. For either party to seek legal recognition of its superior judgment is bound to poison the nearly dry well of trust between the child's personal and medical caregivers.

Substantial differences in their conceptions of the child's welfare already provided ample grounds for distrust between parents and physicians in paediatric medicine. Specialists frequently take it upon themselves to make decisions unilaterally, thereby reducing any residual basis for trust (Magnet and Kluge, 1985: 21, 26-31). Parents have experienced a disregard for their judgment in the care of their children, and attribution of base motives, and, frequently, disturbing medical care directed at their offspring. They have heard horror stories of the torture imposed on children by "dedicated medical researchers" (Stinson and Stinson, 1979; Magnet and Kluge, 1985: 15). They may be aware of the incidence of iatrogenic complications from aggressive treatment;[6] or, they may just be suffering from a lack of adequate information (Stinson and Stinson, 1979; Bridge and Bridge, 1981). Whenever the health care providers take up a stance of moral authority and seek to coerce compliance, they further weaken the bonds of trust which underlie good paediatric care.

In other cases, there may be treatment options which the physician in charge does not feel qualified to administer, e.g., home care for a dying child, chemotherapy rather than a surgical approach, or experimental medicine. Parents who perceive the possibility of an alternative which they are discouraged from pursuing will feel distrustful, and the physician may not feel comfortable having her competence questioned. We should reflect on means for rebuilding effective trust, rather than hastening to secure greater power when we identify conflicting attitudes in operation.

Empirical research on non-compliance supports this commitment to focus on building trust. In their important study, *Achieving Patient Compliance*, DiMatteo and DiNicola argue that the relationship between physician and patient is the most important factor in securing patient compliance (DiMatteo and DiNicola, 1982: 84-89; Jonsen, 1979). In fact, they and others who have studied non-compliance argue that it should not be defined judgmentally as a criticism of patients (or parents), but that it be seen as a term identifying a break-down in the quality of the relationship between physician and patient. After all, medical decisions are made on the

---

[6]Even the specialists acknowledge that iatrogenicity is endemic in perinatology (Jonsen and Lister, 1978: 16).

terms and turf defined by medical experts. For good reason, parents feel at a disadvantage in the event of disagreement, and they often feel intimidated; such discomfort does not always result in blind obedience. On this reading, non-compliance retains a negative connotation, but it is not invoked for "blaming the victim," but for signalling to the physician that more must be done to develop a positive working relationship.[7]

Moreover, several recent studies have indicated that patient compliance is not clearly desirable in all cases. While patients' involvement and commitment in their treatment are highly important to the successful outcome of therapy, patients who make independent decisions about their health program, even if that involves direct contradiction of medical advice, are more likely to improve their health status than those who are passive recipients of the doctor's directives (Benfari, Eacker and Stoll, 1981; Cousins, 1979; Howe, 1981). So, from the patients' point of view, health care seems to be an area for a certain degree of what Baier calls "anti-trust."

My view, then, is that paediatric health care workers should consider appealing to legal channels in pursuing treatment for children only if there is evidence that the parents are abusing the child or neglecting to provide the necessities of life. While Canadian law apparently includes medical necessities under that rubric, I suggest that the term be applied conservatively to include only medical care that is clearly needed, i.e., that which is consistent with the child's overall interests, in the full sense. Other avenues for approval are required if the care offered is controversial, either in its medical effectiveness, or in the burden it places on the child, be it physical, social, or emotional. In the latter case, communication should be improved with parents to seek genuine consent on some form of care which will be recognized as involving the child's overall interests. Alternatively, efforts should be made by health personnel and researchers to explore other, more acceptable forms of treatment, e.g., developing blood substitutes for use for children of Jehovah's Witnesses. My discussion has focused on

---

[7]It is interesting to note that physicians tend to significantly underestimate the degree of mistrust patients feel towards them. They tend to think their own patients are far more appreciative of their efforts, and more compliant than patient data indicate (Darling, 1977; DiMatteo and DiNicola, 1982: 10-12).

dealing with life-threatening conditions, because I think they provide the strongest grounds for appealing to judgments of neglect. In less desperate circumstances, a question of neglect would probably be even harder to support.

If our interest is in addressing cases of neglect, we will refrain from extending the concept to support power struggles between different caregivers. Value disputes over a child's interests ought to be addressed in non-adversarial (non-legalistic) ways.

REFERENCES

Ackerman, Terrence F. 1980. The limits of beneficence: Jehovah's Witnesses and childhood cancer. *The Hastings Center Report* 10 (4): 17-18.

Badley, Robin F. 1984. *Sexual Offenses Against Children*. Ottawa: Canadian Government Publishing Centre.

Baier, Annette. 1985. What do women want in a moral theory? *Nous* 19 (1): 53-63.

Baier, Annette. 1986. Trust and anti-trust. *Ethics* 96: 231-260.

Benfari, R. C., E. Eacker, and J. G. Stoll. 1981. Behavioral interventions and compliance to treatment regimes. *Annual Review of Public Health* 2: 438-439.

Bridge, Paul and Maryls Bridge. 1981. The brief life and death of Christopher Bridge. *The Hastings Center Report* 11 (6): 17-19.

Canadian Family Law Guide. Volume 2. 1985. CCH Canadian Limited.

Cohen, Stuart J. 1979. *New Directions in Patient Compliance*. Lexington, Mass.: Lexington Books.

Cousins, Norman. 1979. *Anatomy of an Illness as Perceived by the Patient: Reflections on Healing and Regeneration.* New York: W. W. Norton and Co.

Darling, Rosalyn Benjamin. 1977. Parents, physicians, and spina bifida. *The Hastings Center Report* 8 (4): 10-14.

Dickens, Bernard M. 1984. Medicine and the law: Withholding paediatric medical care. *The Canadian Bar Review* 62: 196-210.

DiMatteo, M. Robin and D. Dante DiNicola. 1982. *Achieving Patient Compliance: The Psychology of the Medical Practitioner's Role.* New York: Pergamon Press: 84-89, 251.

Gordis, Leon. 1979. Conceptual and methodological problems in measuring patient compliance. *Compliance in Health Care*, edited by R. Brian Haynes, D. Wayne Taylor and David L. Sackett. Baltimore: Johns Hopkins University Press.

Howe, Herbert. 1981. *Do Not Go Gentle*. New York: W. W. Norton and Co.

Jonsen, Albert R. and George Lister. 1978. Newborn intensive care: The ethical problems. *Hastings Center Report* 8 (1).

Jonsen, Albert R. 1979. Ethical issues in compliance. *Compliance in Health Care*, edited by R. Brian Haynes, D. Wayne Taylor, and David L. Sackett. Baltimore: The Johns Hopkins University Press: 113-120.

Magnet, Joseph E. and Eike-Henner W. Kluge. 1985. *Withholding Treatment from Defective Newborn Children.* Cowansville, Quebec: Brown Legal Publications, Inc.

Noddings, Nel. 1984. *Caring*. Berkeley: University of California Press.

Pratt, L. V. 1982. Reshaping the consumer's posture in health care. *Achieving Patient Compliance: The Psychology of the Medical Practitioner's Role*, edited by M. Robin DiMatteo and D. Dante DiNicola. New York: Pergamon Press: 251.

Roueche, Berton. 1986. Annals of medicine: The dinosaur collection. *The New Yorker* (May 12): 102-111.

Russell, Diana E. H. 1986. *The Secret Trauma: Incest in the Lives of Girls and Women*. New York: Basic Books, Inc.

Sherwin, Susan. 1984-1985. A feminist approach to ethics. *Dalhousie Review* 64 (4): 704-713.

Sherwin, Susan. Forthcoming. *In vitro* fertilization: A feminist perspective.

Stinson, Robert and Peggy Stinson. 1979. On the death of a baby. *Atlantic Monthly* (July) 244: 64-72.

The Globe and Mail. 1987. (April 25): A3.

Synthesis: The Larger Perspective
Herbert O'Driscoll

If there is one thing you cannot do in the late twentieth century it is to get a synthesis of anything. First of all I want to say that we have come so far so fast in what we are trying to do. Let me take you back to a moment in 1968 in the Senate hearings which were then trying to establish a National Advisory Commission in the United States on health science in society. It is always interesting to get very prominent people making glib prophecies in which they are proved to be very wrong. There were two very high profile people there at the time in 1968. One was Arthur Cornberg, geneticist, a Nobel Prize winner. The other was Christian Barnard fresh from his triumphs in human heart surgery. Arthur Cornberg said this: "In my judgment no new ethical or moral problems arise from developments in my field. The only use of a commission would be the education of the public on the need for more money for scientific research." The second quote is from Christian Barnard, a shorter one, but no less arrogant: "If non-medical people are to influence medical or scientific policies the results can only be repressive."

A huge change has brought us together, a huge change in the way that Western society thinks and it has happened in our lifetime. Life for all of us has become holistic and feminine. Those are two huge words which constantly we use in too small a way. Somebody has said recently that it may well be that as people look back on the twentieth century, the word "feminist" will have become as significant as words like Aristotelian and Platonist and Thomist were in past generations. We do not know that yet, but it may be.

What do I mean then by holistic? In 1970 two of us stood on the moon, technologically clad to allow us to survive. Just before we came home, we threw out about a dozen sets of Hasselbad cameras, which still lie in the Sea of Tranquillity by the way, to make room for the moon rocks we had gathered. But one of us, just before getting back into the machine, on a kind of afterthought, picked up one of the Hasselbad cameras, pointed it at the jagged horizon of the moon, and waited. Up over that horizon came the loveliest thing that human eyes have ever seen. We saw the totality of things for the first time. We had imagined it, we had written poetry about it, we had painted pictures. But we saw totality for the first time. That has become, apart altogether from being a religious icon, deeply symbolic of a whole new way of thinking.

There are many things you and I could say about that, but let me share four ways in which life has become more holistic. (I hesitate to use the word at all because it is overused and has a lunatic fringe application.) First, on a seasonal level. In the medical world, I know that unless my doctor is a total antiquarian and obscurantist, that I am no longer merely the appendectomy in room three, fourth floor, bed by the window. I have become a sensitive and complex interfacing of body, mind, soul, psyche, whatever. I have become a kind of unity rather than many modules.

Secondly, in terms of our sexuality, we are realizing that within the mystery of our humanity there are two mysteries called femininity and masculinity, and that these are really one spectrum within every single one of us whether we are primarily embodied male or female. Sexuality is becoming regarded more holistically.

Thirdly, it has become a cliché to say that every single economy on this planet, no matter how we label it or attach a philosophy to it or give it a history, is now totally interdependent.

Finally, it has become almost a cliché to say that the relationship between our humanity and the rest of the created order will never again be the same. We are thinking ecologically. We are beginning to think ecosystematically. All these things are something of what I mean when I say that Western consciousness has begun to think holistically, and that is part of the reason why we are interested in these topics.

It has been very hard for us to assemble over the last 300 years. Ironically for 3000 years before that it would have been very simple for us to assemble together as human beings. There are all sorts of people smiling from previous millennia at us and saying: "Well, it has taken you a while to join together as religion, medicine, science, but at least you are here."

Every one of us who was brought up in Western society is basically a child of the last 300 years of the Western world. About 300 years ago, we went out looking for a way to know and we found it. We found a box that said: "This is the way to know" and inside, when we opened the box, there were three things: analysis, reasoning and deduction. They gave us the ability to cut up the universe of thought into information and the physical universe into technology. They gave us endless information and they appealed very strongly to the left side of our brain and the masculine way of dealing with reality. Analysis, reason and deduction, via information and technology, via the left side of our brain and the masculine strengths of our humanity brought us to a place that I will image by calling it the "laboratory." I am not sneering at it; we have done tremendous things over 300 years in the laboratory. But about half way through the twentieth century we became dissatisfied in the laboratory. Something was going wrong. Something was unsatisfying. And we said: "We have got to find another way of knowing." We went over to the old box that we dug up in the late seventeenth century. The lettering on it had changed, rather like the lettering on the end of the pig house in Orwell's *Animal Farm*, which had begun by saying "all pigs are equal" but soon began to say "some pigs are more equal than others." The writing on the box in our society no longer said "This is the way to know." When we looked at it in the 60's it said "This is the only way to know." Then we knew we were in trouble because there was something in us longing for another way to know. So we went out of the laboratory and we searched. In fact our children did, and some of those children of the 60's are adults today. It was a very costly crusade and a very painful one. It involved places like 4th Avenue in Vancouver, Haight Ashbury, Yorkville, and the communes in the valleys of British Columbia. It was a costly children's crusade because what they were trying to find was a very powerful thing. Eventually they found a box and it said: "Here is another way to know which you have forgotten." In the box were three things: synthesis, intuition and imagination. They did not give us more information. They gave us a longing for wisdom about three things: ourselves, relationships and the earth. Synthesis, intuition and imagination via the longing for wisdom about ourselves, about relationships and about the earth, using the right side of our brain and the feminine way of coming at reality, brought us to a place that I will image as the "garden" or "the sacred grove."

Now one of the reasons we are exploring these things is that we have got to put together the sacred grove and the laboratory. We have got to put together the organic and the organization. We have got to put together caring and curing. We have got to put together software and hardware. We have got to put together reflection and action. We have got to think and we have got to feel. For the rest of our lives we will be putting these things together. It has taken us a long time but at least we have begun to come home.

Here we are slugging away in hospitals and universities and at conferences, a congregation of doctors, ethicists, nurses, philosophers, lawyers and clergy. Let me say about half a dozen quick things concerning that coming together. One, it is a very uneasy relationship. Sometimes we see each other with resentment. We see each other as interfering with the smooth goings on of each other's lives. We are all caught in a reality, which I think Pierre Trudeau defined about half way through the 1970's. He said: "What is getting to us is that we used to have the luxury of thinking our way into new ways of acting, and now we have to act our way into new ways of thinking." That is provoking tremendous strain in the interrelationships between all of our disciplines.

Two, we are very often, in the strain of our lives, seeing the worst of each other and thinking the worst of each other. Very often the ethics enterprise is seen as remote, abstract and, at worst, irrelevant. Very often the technology of medicine is seen as pragmatic, impatient, ambitious, impersonal, and, at worst, brutal. Religion is sometimes seen as pathetic, vestigial, primitive and, at worst, neurotic. Law is sometimes seen as self-seeking and, at worst, predatory. Those are the worst visions that we sometimes have of one another.

Three, there is a tremendous cost in time and energy to the holistic view of life for which we are trying to find an interdisciplinary expression. The fact of the matter is that ethics has an ever-expanding agenda. There is personal agenda, lifestyle agenda, familial agenda, social agenda, even political agenda, in terms of such things as distribution of resources.

Four, ethics itself exists in a pluralistic culture. For instance, there is a humanist basis for ethics and there is a religious basis for ethics. Within each of these there are many compartments. Within the religious, in the Western world, you are mainly in a Christian and Jewish ethical system. Within these there are many compartments including Catholic, Protestant, Orthodox and Liberal. That is frustrating at this present stage.

Five, ethics is burdened with imprecision. There is a language in it which is a very imprecise language, "quality of life," "best interest," "ordinary means," "extraordinary means," "autonomy," "beneficence"; these are words that you know better than I. The imprecision of these words is part of our agony but also part of our freedom as well. Ethics is still an art rather than a science. But then one of the new things in my lifetime is that the sciences are facing a new unpredictability and randomness that did not exist even twenty years ago. Medicine itself is full of unpredictability and a new openness. This, of course, is also immensely exciting. Law itself is being forced into new territory where there is no precedent. All I am saying is, we are companions as we face a wilderness. It is not that any one of us holds an infallible wisdom that makes us superior to the rest of us.

Six, ethics is the child of culture and history, therefore, it is highly relative. C. S. Lewis once said that we do not burn old ladies as witches because they live down by the river and keep a black cat. We do not burn them in the 1980's not because we have become more Christian or more charitable or more loving, but because we do not believe they can do the things we used to believe they could do! Yet frequently such people were burned, very ethically, quite regularly. We read of a fourteen-year-old boy in New England being thrashed to death for the good of his soul by a weird cult. There is a long history of that being done very ethically. It was commonplace for the Inquisition in sixteenth-century Spain, on the basis of absolute ethics, to torture and kill. The glories of Greece were given to us on a perfectly ethically based slavery system. It is perfectly possible for us to make a political ethic which would provide an ethical basis for a political dissident to be placed in psychiatric custody. All that needs is an ethic that says that the good of the State is more important than the good of the individual. In other words, the ethic enterprise always needs vigilance and self-criticism because it is always in process. The fact of the matter is that every human discipline in the late twentieth century is in process, including religion.

Finally, in this section, Jean Vanier, founder of the L'Arche movement, a network of communities for mentally handicapped young adults, said of the original house outside Paris: "This is a very human zone, therefore, there are few norms." That statement could be put over the door of ethics conferences because ethics is an enterprise about human life. Even if a complete ethical framework of reference could be constructed , we would still have to apply it with infinite sensitivity to each human situation.

In spite of those limitations, ethical questions are not going to go away. Why? Five quick reasons: (1) The greater the technical resources available to us, the greater the need for ethical reflection about the use of those resources, or, the more cure that is available the more care is necessary. There is a subtle self-cancelling factor that I feel in myself as a human being. The more I know you can do for me medically, the more I fear what you can do to me. (2) That fear and ambivalence about the modern enterprise, part of which is the medical enterprise, could magnify. The relationship between the human and the technical is very fragile in terms of acceptance or rejection. Jonathan Schell (1985), writing in *The New Yorker* in what became a book called *The Fate of the Earth*, has a packed short sentence. Speaking of the essential difference between us and any generation that has gone before us, Schell says that in our day "the human has stepped outside nature and history." He was talking about nuclear technology but we could apply it to medical technology. There is a deep suspicion in our culture, certainly a deep appreciation, but also a fear. It is a mingled thing. There is a feeling that somehow we may have stepped outside nature. You know this and so I need not nag about it.

(3) The new reality that you and I are living in is truly revolutionary,

for the simple reason that the nature that has come under our human dominion is human nature. That has not happened before. For instance, the moment we started into recombinant gene technology we repainted the ceiling of the Sistine Chapel. In the original painting the hand of God is just about to touch and electrify the hand of Adam. Today the divine seems to be saying: "I demand that your hands come into my hand. Together we wield the means to form the future of your own physicality." We are the players and we are the stakes. That is new.

(4) The questions we face are raised by technology and science but they are not technological and scientific questions. They are moral, political, psychological, familial, religious, human questions.

(5) Science cannot, nor at its best does it claim to, tell us what ends we should seek with the tools it gives us. Nor can it tell us how we use its tools without morally violating the human material that we work on.

There are perhaps four or five great new questions our generation faces. The overall one I deliberately put with total simplicity at the risk of being too simple, but this is the way it comes to me as a lay person. The overriding question which applies to almost every facet of late twentieth-century life is: Should we do what we can do? Something that did not hit the news very widely and yet was an extraordinary milestone in the last 300 years of the Western scientific enterprise, happened in 1977. At Asilimar in California the majority of geneticists from the Western world decided by themselves, without government coercion, that they would call a temporary halt to genetic experimentation. It was at that point that the national committees in Japan, Canada, the United States, England, France, etc., were formed. There are voices such as David Suzuki, who feel that the temporary halt was not sufficient. In saying this I am trying to give a slight context to that great overriding question, should we do what we can do?

What is human? I do not have to nag at that question. You ask it in your own minds. In what circumstances does medical intervention violate the purpose and meaning of human life? Towards what kind of life are we pressing? If there is validity in those questions, the dialogue between the disciplines is not going to go away but is going to get more significant. If so, it is absolutely necessary that we accord each other integrity and that we do not go on making stereotypes of one another. I think the struggle not to do that will be most difficult for law and medicine because they have the most power to claw at each other. They have done it in the United States and it is self-defeating to both. From now on, if we are going to exist as intelligent beings, we have to become aware of what I call the Babel factor. Remember the old story about the tower that humanity built? God decided to make all the people speak different languages so that the tower failed. We are all trying to build a tower. At its best it is not an arrogant tower; it is a tower of healing for humanity. But in the last couple of generations we have come to admire specialization so much that if somebody does not understand our language then that person is outside the circle or is irrelevant. All of us, from now on, are going to need built-in translators in our heads, so that, if someone is using a religious language or a psychological language or some other kind of language, we do not dismiss that person but we say: "What in my language is being said?"

The future of the family physician is absolutely imperative, or, if we are not going to use that kind of language, somebody performing as we now understand the family physician to be performing. Why? Because I know very well, as I go into the door of my doctor, that I am not going into two little rooms. I am going into the entrance to an endless and terrifying country. Behind that tiny office there is a maze that takes me to other figures which do not know me and some terrible machines which can tend my body but also terrify my mind. I need a guide in that maze. I need a companion for my journey, and, if we do not understand that, we will create deep alienation in the whole medical enterprise. Let me express it in terms that all of you can identify in some way. As Frodo I need a Gandalf to take me over Rivendell. As Luke Skywalker I need Obiwan Ben Kanobi to take me across that lonely galaxy. As Dante I want my Beatrice to go through the underworld where I have to go sometimes in my illness. As John Bunyon's pilgrim I need Mr. Standfast. As Beowulf I need my friend to take me to the end of the world to find the meaning of life and death. As Hamlet, as I go through my shadows and my fear, I need a Horatio. As Euridice in the underworld of my illness I need an Orpheus. And that relationship is going to get even more necessary.

Religion, in the Western hemisphere, now seems vestigial. However, it may be changing before our eyes, and it may, as it has already in Islam, become something so new to us that it boggles our mind. It might in fact become something extremely unpleasant. Why? We live in an apocalyptic history. That is a time of vast change, turmoil, threat, fear, anxiety, promise and hope. If you could sit down and talk to anybody from the fifth century around the Mediterranean or the fourteenth century in Europe, they would know exactly what you were talking about because they felt it. Let me give you an image from an ancient book which we tend to dismiss. Somebody has a dream and in this dream he sees a woman against the background of the universe. The sun and the moon and the stars revolve around her head. She is pregnant, and in front of her there is a dragon waiting to devour the child. This is an image of an apocalyptic history. There has never been a time when civilization has been more pregnant with possibility of every single kind than in our lifetime. Yet there is the dragon who waits to devour. One aspect of the dragon is the nuclear dragon. There are others; the population dragon, the pollution dragon; there are many dragons. Because of this there are always certain things taking place in the human psyche in an apocalyptic history. It is happening all around us, it is sitting with a thousand psychosomatic symptoms in physicians' waiting rooms. It is the fact that there is a tremendous sense of awe from the nature of the times people are living in. Awe is a mixture of wonder and terror, and what always happens from that mixture is an explosion of spirituality. The trouble is, we tend to think of spirituality as a nice thing. It is not. It is a total spectrum. What do we mean by spirituality? There is a feeling in the late twentieth century among people that has nothing to do with whether or not they darken the door of places like churches. It is a feeling that the meaning of human experience and human existence is not merely within that experience and that existence. If you examine that you are talking about the beginnings of spirituality. However, there is a dark side to it. There is a total spectrum of contemporary spiritual experience. It goes from the irrational and the superstitious, the neurotic and the psychotic, right up to the mystical, the liberating and the self-sacrificial. Two great contemporory psychological and spiritual archetypes are Jim Jones, psychotic in the jungles of Guyana, and

Mother Theresa in an urban jungle called Calcutta, totally self-sacrificial and liberating.

For such reasons religion is no longer merely residual in Western culture. The reason that religion is not residual in Western culture anymore is what we call modernity. Modernity is the whole interplay of the technical, the pluralistic, the secular and the urban, all of which creates the culture that you and I take totally for granted. Remember however that modernity is very recent; and it is very ambiguous. It is only an experiment and there is arising a tremendous ambivalence towards it. If its human costs are too great, and they are getting very great, there will be a revulsion against it, as has already happened in Islam, particularly in Iran, and of which there are signs among millions of people in the United States. Religion has a dual side. If we crush the healthy one we will get the dark side. Healthy religion needs to be catholic, meaning that it has room for all facets of existence; sacramental, joining the physical and the intangible; liberal, having a deeply human and feminine element, affirming the insights of other disciplines in the world. The dark side of religion can be deeply paternalistic; at worst, totalitarian, anti-intellectual and anti-technical. If you want to get a glimpse of that world as it comes into the imagination of the artist today, pick up Margaret Atwood's (1985) story of *The Handmaid's Tale*. In other words, there is a dark side of religion that rejects the world and it rejects culture.

Religion then is not going to go away. It is not going to go away from our patients. It is not going to go away from the ultimate questions that people are asking, nor from the ultimate moments of their lives such as illness and death. Therefore, it is becoming terribly important for any professional today not to be under the illusion that religion is a kind of pathetic memory which is vestigial to the modern world. Instead we had better get to know its reality. We had better give it validity and we had better not dismiss it because we may get something much worse in its place.

To end, what good things have we discovered? I think we have discovered that life is returning to being tremendously collegial, communal and interdisciplinary. That can only be good, frustrating as it is sometimes.

Secondly, we are realizing that we are no longer modules in a machine but cells in a body.

Thirdly, we are moving from seeing reality as subject/object to being subject/subject, and that is a huge change in Western consciousness. We are beginning to realize that the earth, for instance, is not a scientific experiment from which our humanity is separated in some lordly way, but we are realizing, as an American poet has said, "that the world is a wedding."

A lot of people have been saying that for a long time, including native spirituality, which we dismissed as ancient and primitive, only to turn around to find it waiting for us to catch up with it. It was also said, very loudly, by Franciscan spirtuality, by Eastern Orthodox spirituality, by ancient Celtic spirituality, but all that is a whole other story. All I am emphasizing is that we in the West have come back to something that others did not forget but we did.

Fourth, we are realizing the uniqueness of persons. I know it sounds a cliché but it may be our greatest achievement.

Fifth, we are realizing that the more we can help one another to live the more we must help one another to die. We are also realizing something that I remember Rollo May saying some years ago in a symposium in Vancouver, where he said: "There will always be the professionals but in the next couple of decades there will come the paraprofessionals, and they have come." He said: "There will always be need for the paraprofessional because the suffering of an apocalyptic time will be too much for the professionals." Then he said:

> Beyond the paraprofessionals we will come to know the truth, that all of us in the late 20th century society have in some sense to become healers, even if we are talking only about the very normal gifts given to everybody, gifts such as touching, sensitizing, laughing, being with, forgiving, listening, etc.

A final quick illustration. Jesus of Nazareth once said that there was a man who sowed wheat in his field, and with the wheat there came up weeds. His servants came to him and said: "Do you want us to rip out the weeds?" He said: "No, because if you rip out the weeds you rip out the wheat. Just leave it to the time of the harvest." What does that story mean? It means that the whole human enterprise will alway be ambiguous. There is never going to be a perfect ethical system. There is never going to be a perfect legal system. There is never going to be a perfect medical system. There is never going to be a perfect religious system, contrary to the illusions of some people. We are all in that ambiguous reality, and we are in it together. That, as they say, is the name of the game. But the fact is that this is the only game in town. That is why we have to play it together, carefully, thoughtfully, faithfully.

REFERENCES

Atwood, Margaret. 1985. *The Handmaid's Tale.* Toronto, Canada: McClelland and Stewart.

Schell, Jonathan. 1985. *The Fate of the Earth.* New York: Alfred Knopf.

INDEX